THE COMPLETE GUIDE TO
SHORT BOARD SAILING

THE COMPLETE GUIDE TO
SHORT BOARD
SAILING

Jeremy Evans

Foreword by Robby Naish
Photographs by Alex Williams

INTERNATIONAL MARINE PUBLISHING COMPANY
Camden, Maine

The Complete Guide to Short Board Sailing
was conceived, edited, designed and
produced by Holland & Clark Limited

Artist
Nicolas Hall

Designer
Julian Holland

Editors
Philip Clark
Christine McMullen

Design Assistant
Martin Smillie

Library of Congress Cataloging-in-Publication Data
Evans, Jeremy.
  The complete guide to short board sailing.
  1. Windsurfing. I. Title
GV811.63.W56E82   1987   797.3'3   86-20095
ISBN 0-87742-245-1

Phototypeset in Great Britain by
Input Typesetting Limited, London

Printed and bound in Hong Kong by
Mandarin Offset

Published by International Marine Publishing Company
21 Elm Street, Camden, Maine 04843

Contents

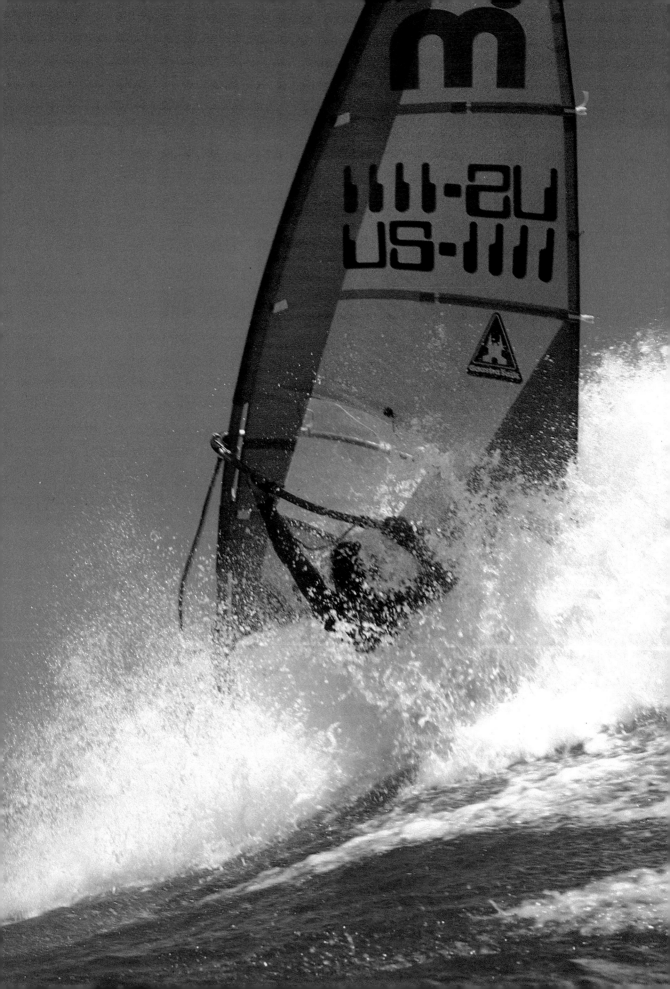

Foreword by Robby Naish

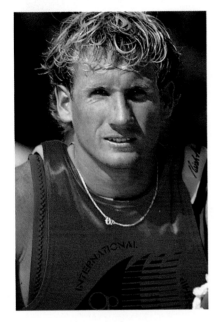

Robby (above and left) is without a doubt the greatest windsurfer and short board sailor there has ever been. He's won every title of note, including taking the World Cup for four years in succession.

For me, short board sailing is by far the most fun and exciting aspect of windsurfing. Raceboards, freestyle, and allround boards are great in small doses, but I could never sail them every day – not anymore – not after the evolution of the short board. Windsurfers can now jump higher, ride bigger waves, and sail faster than any other sailing vessels in history.

Short board sailing is addicting. Around the world on almost every lake and ocean, people are riding them. All it takes is 12 knots of wind or more – enough to plane, and you're on your way.

You don't have to be a great sailor to sail a short board. In fact, here in Hawaii a lot of people learn on them, never touching anything over ten feet long. If you can waterstart, you can ride one – if you can't – get out there and learn – you don't know what you're missing.

The important thing, whether you are sailing in waves or on flat water, sailing in five knots on a production board, or in thirty knots on a custom Naish Hawaii board, is to have fun.

Enjoy yourself – whatever level you're sailing at.

aloha,

Robby Naish

Short Boards in Action

Alex Williams has taken most of the photos in this book, while others have been provided by Stuart Sawyer. The dramatic shots in this section show short boards in action.

Alex first became a surfer in 1973. He developed an interest in photography and made the transition from surfer to becoming Europe's leading in-water surf photographer.

Camera Gear
The tools of Alex's trade are Canon Fls with motordrives which are capable of shooting five frames per second: lenses ranging from 17 mm ultrawide to 800 mm telephoto; and custom-built Scott Preiss glassfibre/Plexiglass housings. He uses Kodachrome film exclusively.

Favourite Locations
Alex's travels take him around the world from his home base in the UK's West Country to the major surf locations in Europe, Hawaii, the West Indies and Australia.

He rates the UK as the toughest venue – it's cold, there are fierce currents, and the weather never behaves to order. Understandably his favourite location is Hawaii – ideal conditions and many excellent sailors who can perform to order in front of the camera.

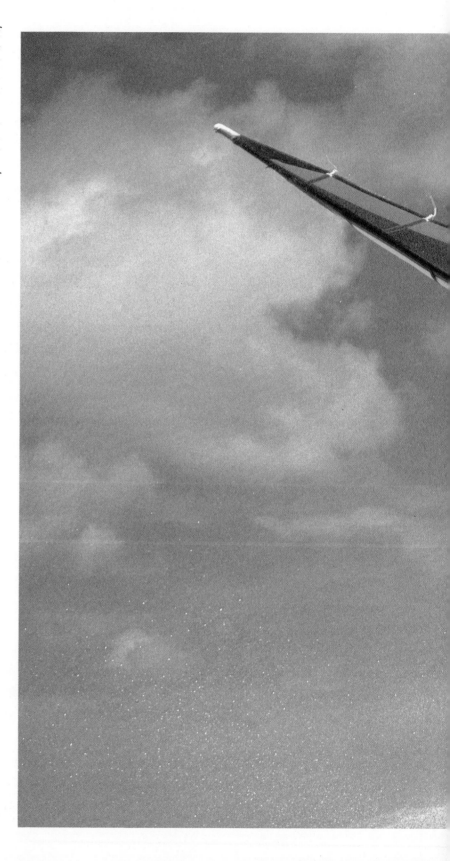

Right: Angus Chater about to attempt a vertical landing (!) off Diamond Head in Hawaii. Angus worked closely with Alex over a number of years. They became a skilful team, with maximum output and minimum danger for either party.

In-water surf photography of this type is physically demanding and can be dangerous. There are big waves, cold, and boards zipping past the lens at 30 knots.

With his surfing background and superb fitness Alex is well able to survive!

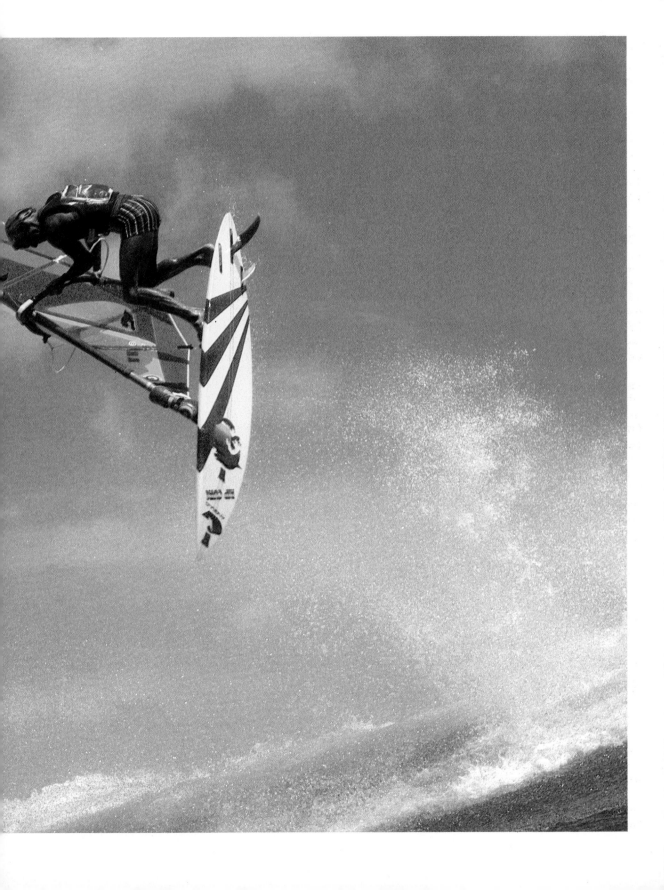

The King in Action

This is the King of Windsurfing, Robby Naish, riding along a wall of white water off Hookipa in Hawaii.

Robby started winning windsurfing championships when he was 13, and has continued through 10 years of competition. He has won every kind of event from long board racing to wave performance.

There are maybe a handful of wavesailors of the same calibre as Robby, with fellow Hawaiians Pete Cabrinha and Craig Masonville leading contenders for his title. No one would argue, however, that Robby is unmatched today as the greatest allrounder windsurfing has ever seen.

Robby's principal sponsors are Mistral and Gaastra. He has raced and performed in wave events for them for many years and, together with his father Rick Naish, has developed many of Mistral's prototype and production boards under the 'Naish Hawaii' label. All the Naish boards are designed and shaped by Rick and Harold Iggey in Kailua on the main Hawaiian island of Oahu, and their best known production designs include the Mistral Diamond Head and Hookipa.

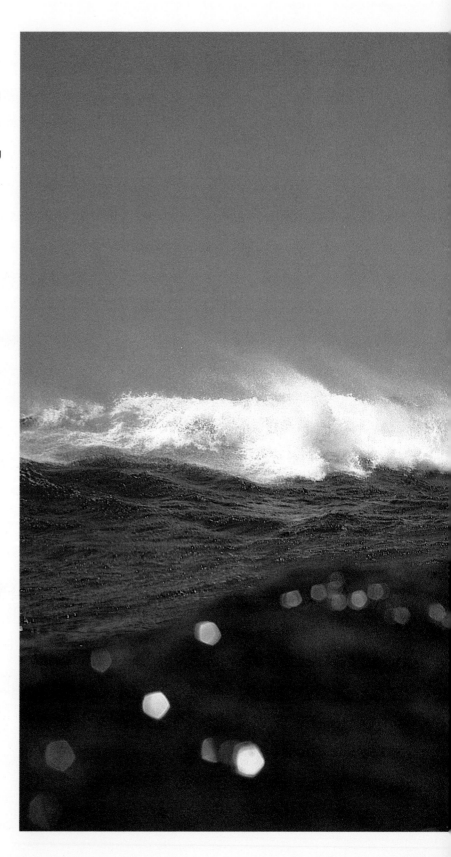

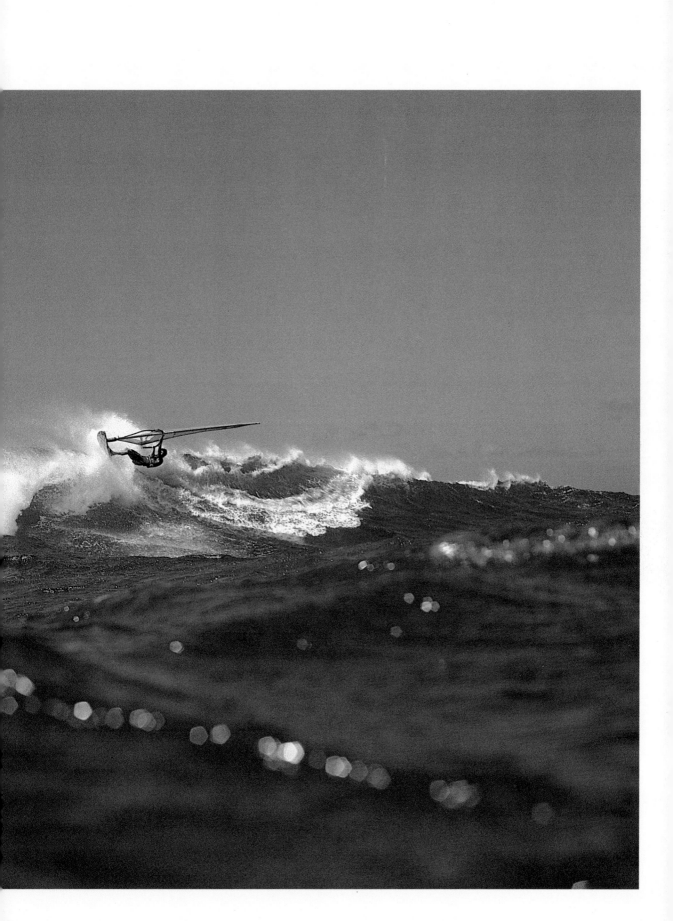

Off the Wall!
English rider Gary Gibson about to take off while riding a wave at Cotillo, a premier short board location on the island of Fuerteventura in the Canaries.

There is more information about Fuerteventura on page 128 – it's rated as an excellent spot for European short board sailors as it is easily accessible and provides a good place for winter breaks.

Like all sailors trying to make a living out of windsurfing, Gary knows how to provide the photographer with the maximum dramatic display for each shot. Here he gives a full frontal close-up to the camera before blasting past Alex Williams in the water.

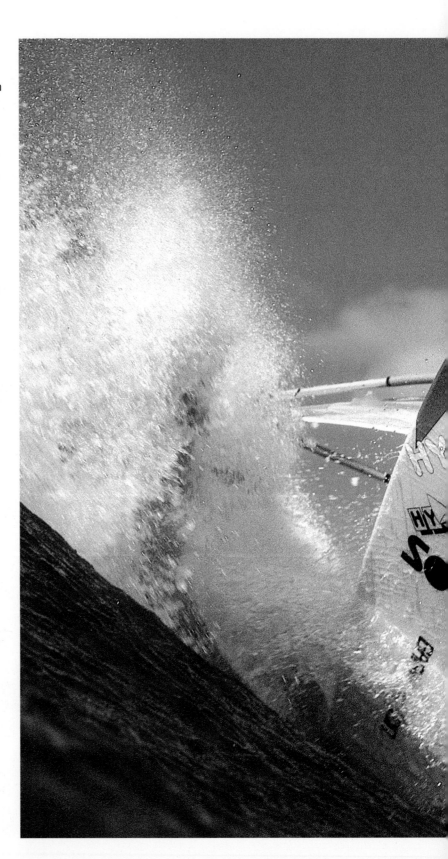

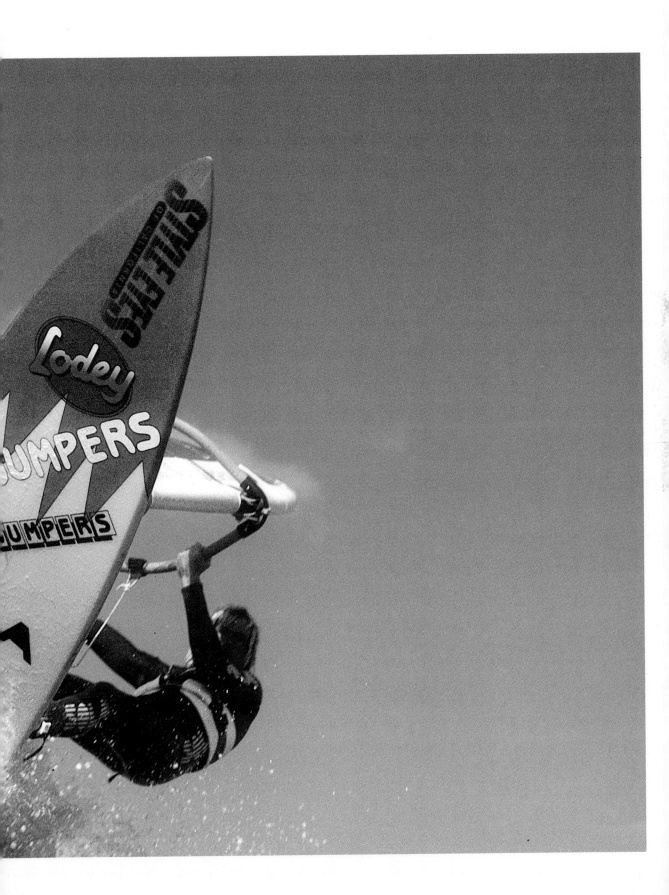

Jumping Jack Flash

Stuart Sawyer leaps to order off the beach at Matagorda on the island of Lanzarote in the Canaries.

Stuart is a professional windsurfer who has made a good living out of sponsorship. Born in England, he first went to live in Hawaii in 1983, where his romance with local windsurfer Debbie Floreani also blossomed into a useful windsurfing promotions partnership.

Stuart and Debbie have worked with many major manufacturers and sponsors both in and out of windsurfing. These have included Sailboard, Vitamin Sea, Tushingham, Gul and Nabisco. Their job is to bring those companies as much exposure as possible, and they achieve this by making sure they get the best photos of the company logos in action, and that those photos are widely published.

You will see Stuart's photos popping up throughout this book, as he shows off his expertise with such techniques as the helicopter tack, donkey kick, aerial gybe, and other specialities.

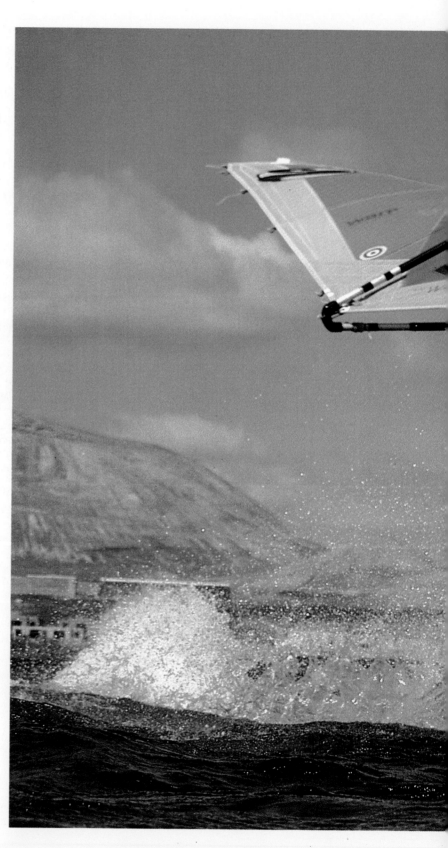

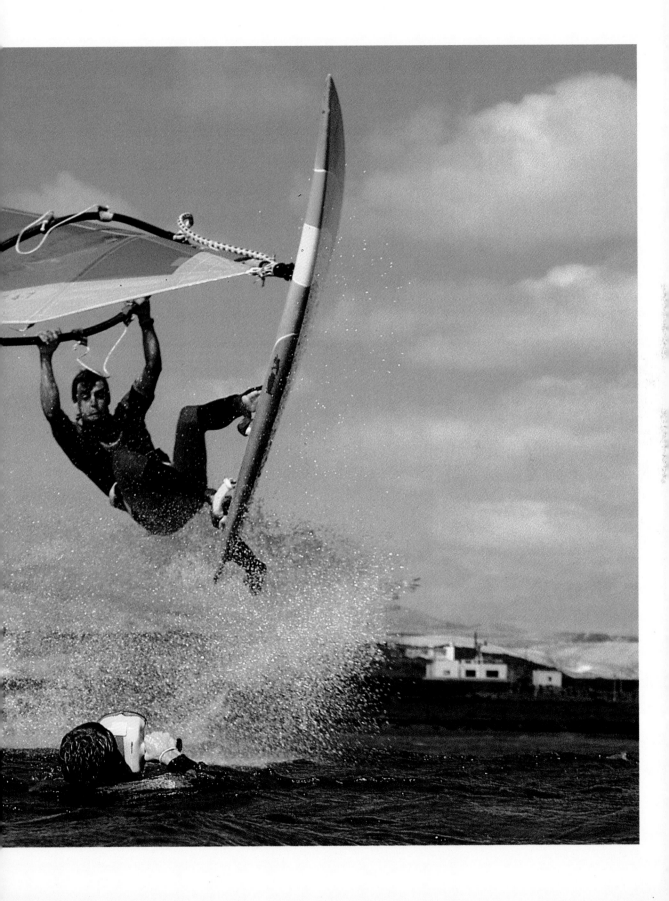

Night Time Images

Alex Williams gets a double take of Angus Chater night sailing in Kailua Bay. Getting this picture just right took a lot of experimental late night sessions for sailor and photographer, both of whom were well aware of the possibility of sharks – watch out for those dark shapes lurking beneath the surface!

Angus rated these sessions as a valuable test of the senses and co-ordination. Gybing while being unable to see the booms had to be instinctive and accomplished by feel alone. With no visual distractions he discovered he could gauge the gybe perfectly, and accomplish it faster and more successfully than he could in broad daylight.

NB Short board sailing by night is not to be recommended at all unless you are an expert. Always take very great care, and ensure that there are people on hand to watch you and help if necessary.

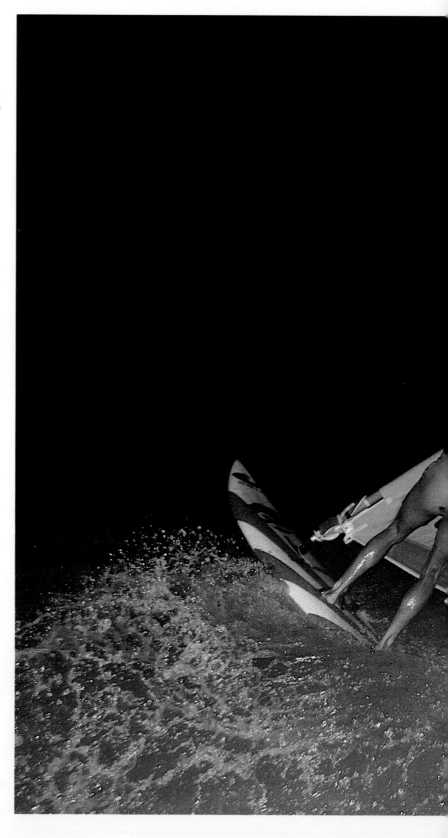

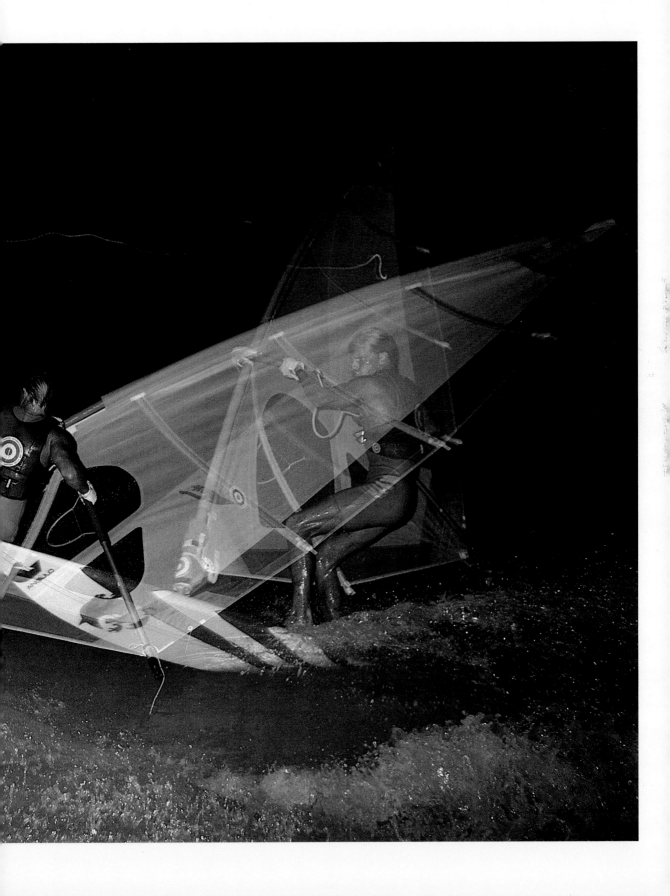

Bird's Eye View

This is what it looks like sailing a 295 – the view is from the top of the mast. Stuart Sawyer is batting along, and if you look closely you will see his left hand is squeezing the button connected to the remote control camera attached to the mast top. To allow for spray and wipeouts the camera, of course, has to be equipped with a waterproof housing.

The 295 is the most popular type of short board. With plenty of volume it performs successfully in a wide range of conditions from Force 3 upwards – and if the sailor hasn't mastered the waterstart it can usually be uphauled if necessary.

The Sailboard 295 which Stuart is riding is a swallowtail (for width and stability) designed by Brian Hinde, one of the Hawaiian shapers.

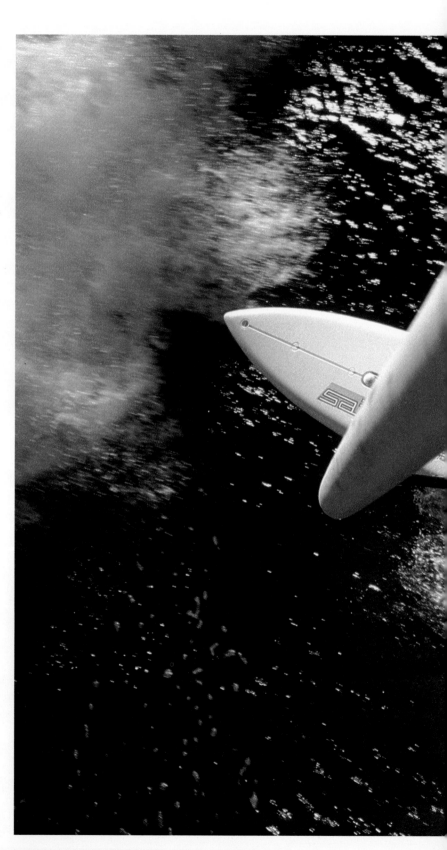

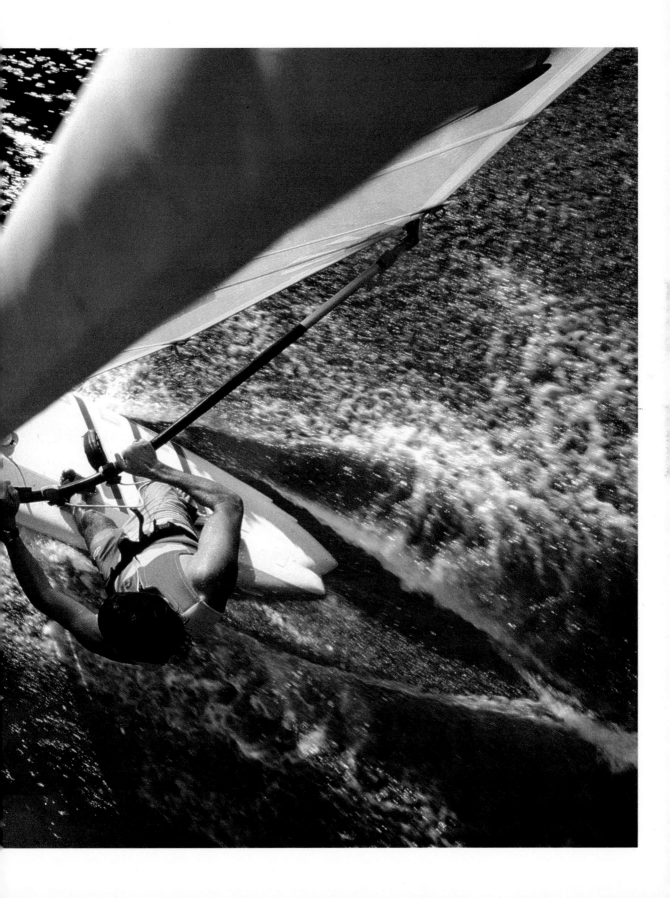

Upside Down! Inside Out!
At the highest level, the short board
sailor has to be a skilled athlete with
the abilities of a contortionist and
gymnast. In this photo Angus Chater
gets all twisted up on his way down
from a sky-high jump off Diamond
Head, Oahu.

Excellent technique must be
combined with the necessary degree
of physical fitness, and in this top
league of the sport accidents are
always a possibility – sprains and
broken bones are the not infrequent
results of too many heavy landings.
The most important safety factor is
the bale-out. When the sailor decides
he is losing control, he must get
away from the board and rig to make
sure that he doesn't crash land on it
– or vice versa, which can be even
more disastrous.

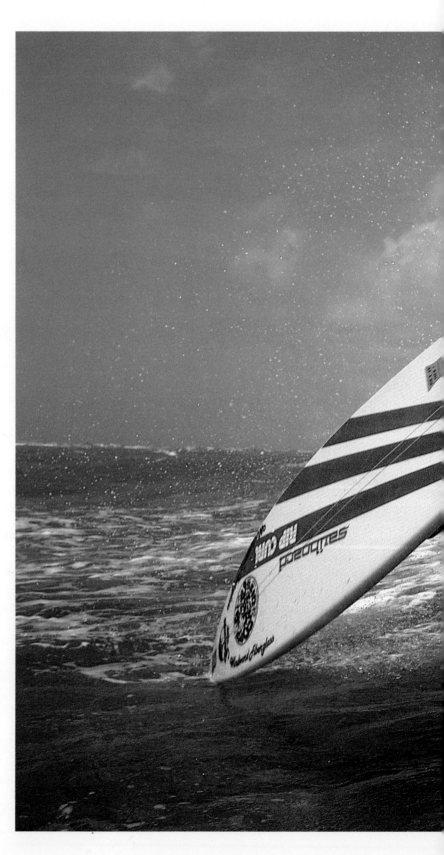

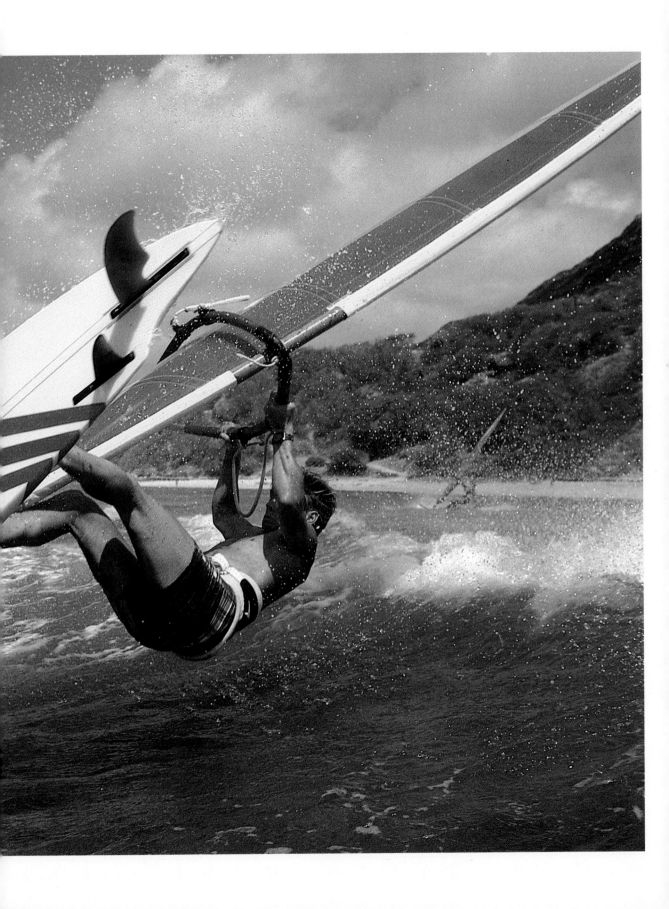

**Underwater Waterstart – or
Underwater Jump?**
This is what a windsurfing
photographer gets up to when he's
on location and finds that the wind
conditions are hopeless for sailing.

The sailor is Gary Gibson, and
both he and Alex Williams are
underwater off the island of
Fuerteventura, in the Canaries, during
a spell of winter training.

It's always a case of being
adaptable and creative if you want the
profession to pay – there are plenty
of windsurfing photographers, and
they're all trying to come up with
something that is spectacular – or
just different!

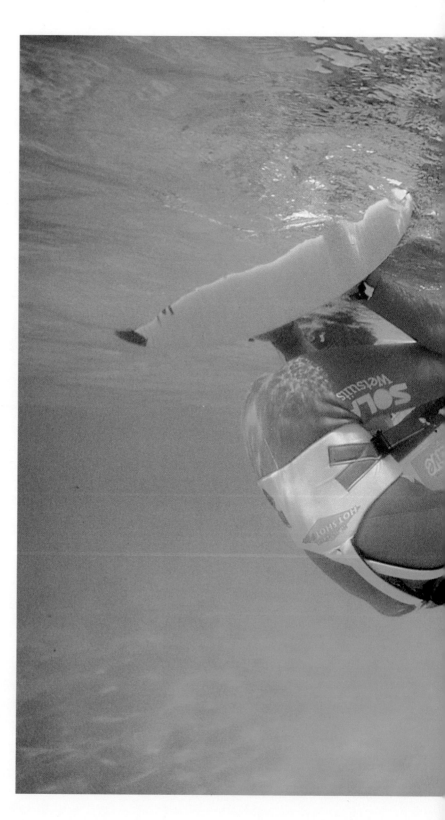

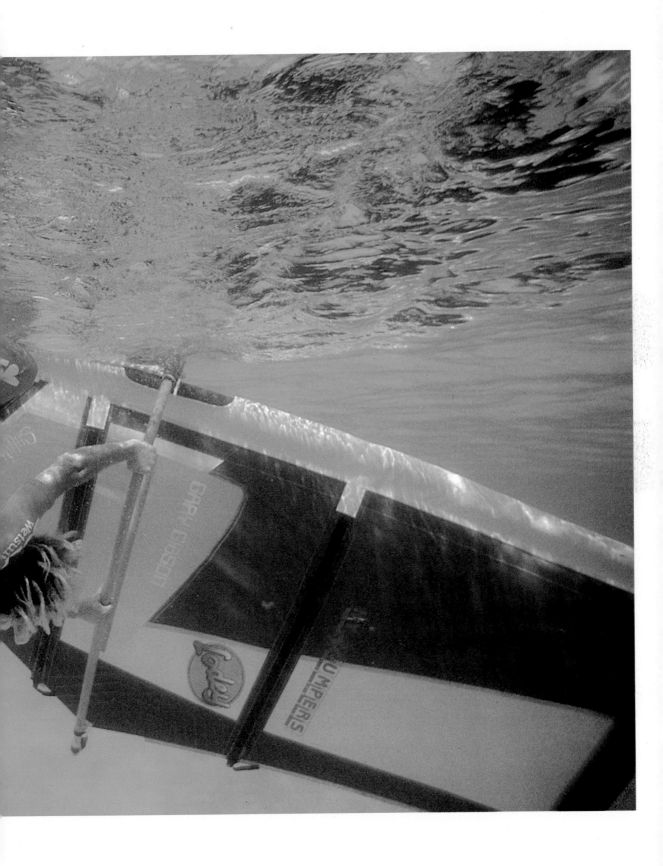

Evolution of the Short Board

In the beginning was the Windsurfer – the original windsurfing board which was based on a big, long Malibu-style surfboard. The Windsurfer caught on fast in Europe, where prevailing light to moderate winds made it an ideal board and easy to handle.

Meanwhile a few Windsurfers were being sailed in Hawaii, where the predominant big waves and strong winds made it very difficult to handle. As a result footstraps were developed, plus the harness as pioneered by Larry Stanley around 1978; and a special kind of strong wind Windsurfer called the Rocket was designed.

Strong Wind Competitions
By 1980 the most exciting, top league windsurfing competition was the Pan Am Cup, held off Kailua in Hawaii during March. This was the first strong wind, funboard style competition, with long races through the swells and 'ins-and-outs' through the surf – the forerunners of modern slalom style competition.

Early boards were hard to control, both on the wave and airborne, so they started to be made shorter, capitalizing on the score or so of Hawaiian surfboard shapers who could produce a custom windsurfer to order in a matter of days. Many of these early experiments were awful designs (wide, high volume tails were the norm), but they were part of a rapid development.

Immediately after the 1980 Pan Am Cup, Hoyle Schweitzer staged the Maalaea Speed Trials on the island of Maui. Many of the boards used could be described as weird and wonderful! A design breakthrough occurred when Hugh England of Windsurfing Hawaii did what with hindsight seems so obvious – he simply added a windsurfing rig to a small, gun style surfboard which has become the normal sinker in use today.

The First Sinker
This, unfortunately, was far in advance of the current sailors' windsurfing skills for, although waterstarts were part of the freestyle repertoire, they were not sufficiently developed. However, Hugh had shown the way, and he was soon followed by Matt Schweitzer (Hoyle's son) and Mike Waltze.

In Europe, however, these advances were only glimpsed when Jürgen Hönscheid broke the record at the Weymouth Speed Trials in September 1981.

The Short Board Explosion
From then on short board manufacture really took off. The custom builders who had made a quiet living from surfboards were deluged with orders for windsurfers, and some of them moved into making glassfibre moulded 'pop outs' in order to keep the supply up and the prices down.

Essentially, it is the same today. The committed enthusiasts tend to buy custom boards which are widely produced in the USA (mainly in Hawaii and California), Australia, the UK (mainly in the West Country); and to a lesser extent in France, Germany, and other centres with local demand.

The alternative to custom made is a production short board, made by the giants such as Mistral, Tiga and Fanatic; or there is a wider choice from specialist small builders who produce pop out.

Shaper/designers today have star status, and leading lights are Harold Iggey (Naish Hawaii), Jimmy Lewis, Brian Hinde and John Hall.

Design Evolution
Having found out how to sail a small surfboard with a rig, the early designers began to explore the extremes. The most obvious step was to find the minimum length possible, and the hottest

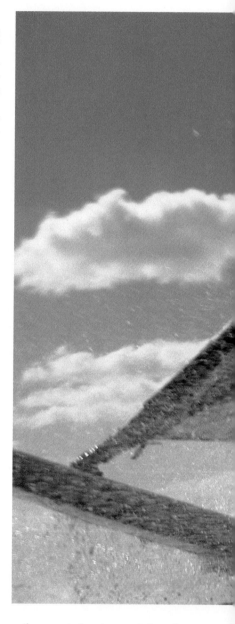

sailors tried sizes right down towards two metres (6 ft 6 in). They realized eventually that the shortest practical length was at least 2.40 m (7 ft 10 in), while the most 'useful' length was closer to three metres (9 ft 10 in).

At the same time they went through all the variations of shape, with complex swallowtails and multi-wingers being accompanied by multi-channel bottoms.

Nowadays much more simple

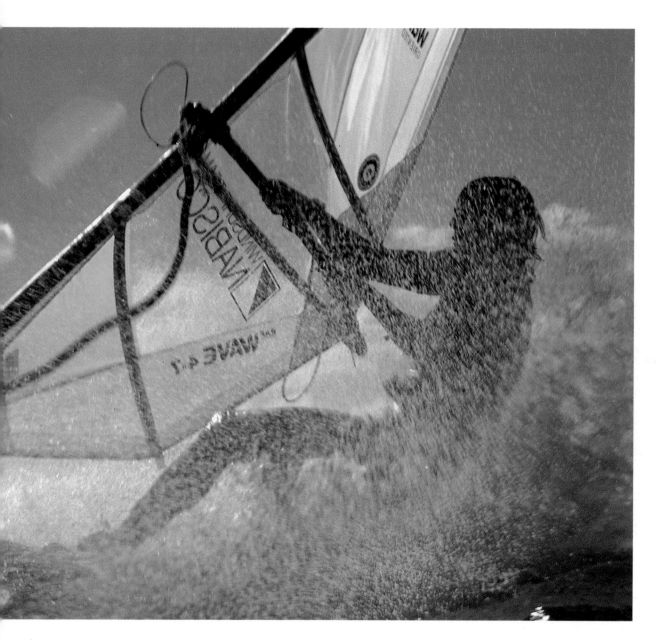

shapes are the norm, as it is now widely accepted that what really matters is rocker line and volume distribution while most of the other design features are just fancy trimmings.

Design has settled down and most future progress is likely to be in small details, as well as in stronger, more durable construction and stiffness.

This is all good news for those who are buying short boards; in the early days the customer was frequently 'experimented upon', but now basic short board design is sound and invariably 'right'.

Rig Evolution

Like the early boards, the first rigs were also pretty primitive. Long booms and flappy, hollow leeches made control a nightmare, and the pioneers struggled to control the boards whilst today's short board sailor can choose from a number

Above: In a surprisingly short time the short board and its rig have evolved into a sophisticated, highly tuned machine.

of first rate rigs.

Virtually all the development work has been done in Hawaii, where the conditions are so ideal that a sailmaker can test a sail in the morning, recut it in the afternoon, and try it again the next day and so on until it's perfect.

Short Boards Today

After much experiment and many extreme designs, today's short boards fall into three main categories – the 295, the 270 and the sinker.

The 295

Most manufacturers have a board in their range which is about 2.95 m long (9 ft 8 in). Volume is usually around 120 litres, which gives enough flotation for uphauling – although the overall size of the board will make it so unstable that waterstarting is always better, and will often be the only way of getting started.

Most contemporary 295s have evolved from World Cup competition slalom events, and consequently many of them are dubbed 'slalom'. This means you can expect a bottom shape with concaves, and a drawn-out tail with a single fin for maximum speed. The board also has manoeuvrability for easy gybes, performs reasonably in waves, and jumps effortlessly.

The 270

A few manufacturers have a board of around 2.70 m (8 ft 10 in) – the smallest board in the range. However, when you get to this more advanced type of short board sailing you may well go for a one-off custom made board – it's hand made, it's exclusive, it looks great, and unfortunately it's very fragile.

With a volume of around 90 litres most boards in this category are marginal floaters so long as you're not too heavy – you can't expect to uphaul, but the board won't sink beneath you when it's stationary. Designs tend to cater either for wavesailing or speed.

The Sinker

For an average weight sailor a true sinker is likely to be less than 80 litres volume, which means that the board will sink until it starts to plane. The market for true sinkers is limited and the majority are, therefore, custom made or manufactured in relatively small numbers.

Uses also tend to be more specialized. For instance, a speed board is a long, drawn-out gun designed purely for flat water speedsailing in minimum winds of Force 5; while a wave board is wider and more floaty, designed for maximum manoeuvrability and acceleration.

Right: Up, up and away! Stuart Sawyer demonstrates the merits of a custom sinker. He is sailing off Matagorda Beach, a favourite venue for Europeans in Lanzarote, Canaries.

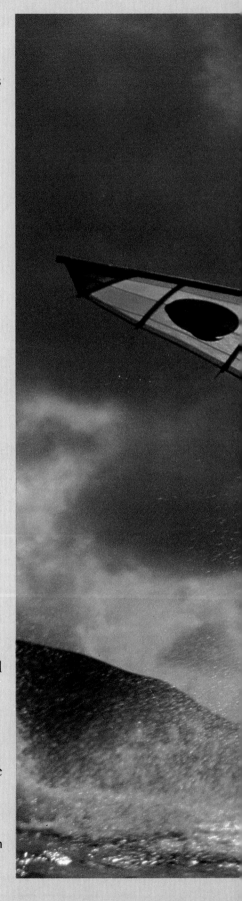

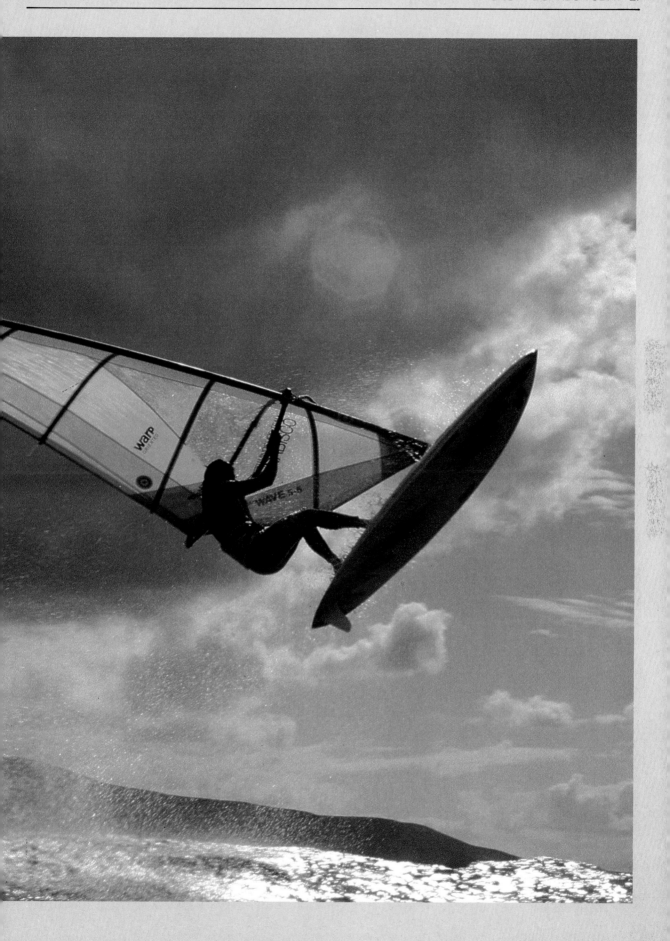

Short Board Design

To the untutored eye all boards may look much the same apart from differences in length, but the short board designer needs to be an expert in compromising between a number of conflicting factors:

* *Volume*
* *Outline and tail shape*
* *Rocker line*
* *Rail shape*
* *Bottom shape*
* *Strap, fin and mast positions*
* *Construction*

Volume

The more volume a board has, the better its performance is likely to be in marginal conditions. So a 295 with 125 litres volume will perform better in Force 4 than a 295 with 100 litres. On the other hand a 100 litre board will become progressively easier to control and faster as the wind grows stronger.

The designer and the sailor must therefore decide whether they are looking for a board which is best in Force 4, 5 or 6. The designs may compromise so that they're good performers in as wide a range of conditions as possible.

Positive Buoyancy

Volume should be seen in terms of positive buoyancy. This determines how well the board will perform in marginal conditions, and how it will support the weight of the sailor – is it a floater, a marginal or a sinker?

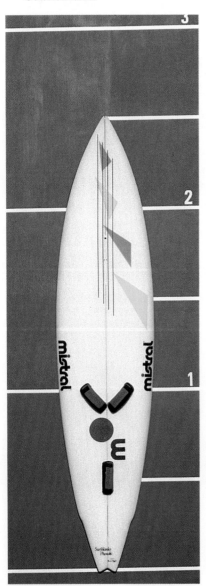

A small 250 with the wide point about mid-way, and three strap layout.

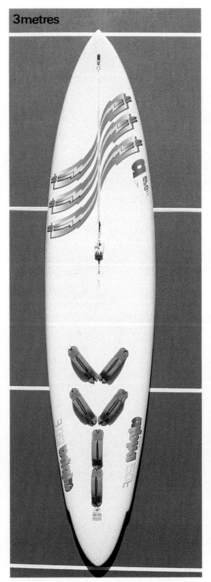

The classic 295 has plenty of volume and width for marginal conditions.

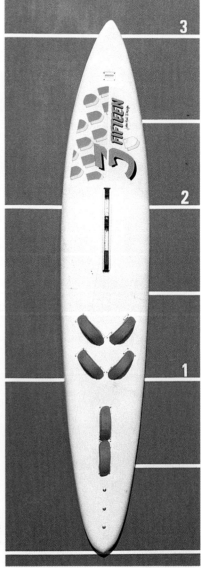

A gun style outline with narrow drawn-out tail.

If you know the board's volume you can calculate positive buoyancy using the following equation:

Board volume	+97 litres
Rig weight	− 6 kg
Board weight	−10 kg
Sailor's weight	−70 kg
Sailor's wetsuit	− 6 kg
Positive Buoyancy	= 5 litres

In this example the five litres positive buoyancy would mean the board was a marginal, needing to be waterstarted at all times, and requiring the top end of Force 4 to reach its full performing potential. If the wind were any less, it could just about be sailed home by an experienced sailor, though if the wind dropped off to below Force 3 he would have great difficulty.

How Much Volume?

If you are unsure what amount of volume you should be looking for, the best advice is that too much is better than too little. With modern construction methods high volume boards can be built very light, and if the rest of the design is right the board should be able to combine high volume with control in a range of conditions.

Guidelines to how much volume is needed by an average weight 70 kg sailor are: 120 litres for a 295 in Force 4; 90 litres for a 270 in Force 5; 80 litres for a sinker in Force 6.

Outline and Tail Shape

Having gone through a period of rapid evolution and development, short board outlines have settled into an accepted pattern with three typical examples shown on the facing page.

Outline is principally governed by the position of the wide point and the tail shape. If the wide point is forward it will promote a long, drawn out tail and a narrow outline which is known as a gun, and is intended for speed.

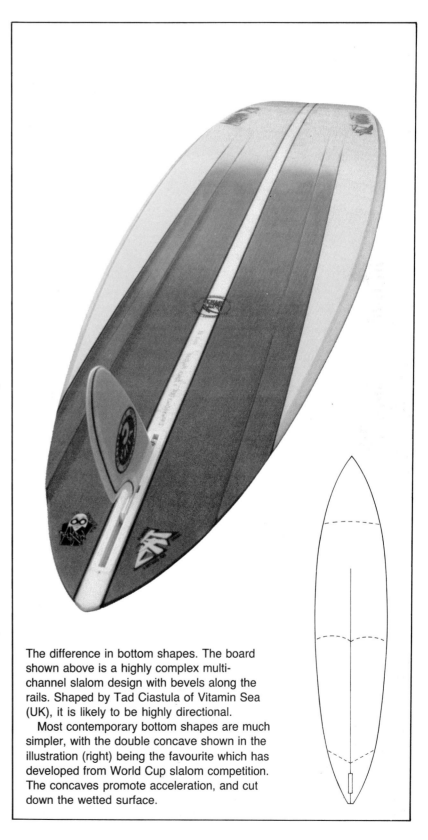

The difference in bottom shapes. The board shown above is a highly complex multi-channel slalom design with bevels along the rails. Shaped by Tad Ciastula of Vitamin Sea (UK), it is likely to be highly directional.

Most contemporary bottom shapes are much simpler, with the double concave shown in the illustration (right) being the favourite which has developed from World Cup slalom competition. The concaves promote acceleration, and cut down the wetted surface.

It is not so suitable for performance in marginal conditions or manoeuvrability, because of the comparatively low volume of the tail area.

Fancy Tails
In the early days of short board design fancy tails were in vogue, with swallowtails, wingers and other trimmings all claimed to make the board looser, faster and better. Now it is generally accepted that it is width and thickness which are most important, and there is a trend towards the simple pintail, occasionally equipped with wingers to give a little extra width if the board seems too narrow.

Wide tails allow the board to pivot easily while narrow tails have more grip on the water. A thick tail won't sink but may 'bounce-out' in a turn when the going gets hairy; a thin tail sinks to give better traction, but will obviously need more drive to make it get up and go.

Rocker Line
All shapers agree that rocker line is critical to performance. Tail rocker, or 'lift', is particularly important for manoeuvrability, since it allows the sailor to pull most of the board clear of the water while it pivots on its tail, with the curve of the rocker helping to dictate the arc of its turn as it banks through a gybe.

In simple terms flat tail rocker equals speed; while plenty of tail rocker equals manoeuvrability.

A compromise is needed which depends on the purpose of the board. For an allround short board you can expect a norm of about three to 3.5 cm (1⅛–1⅜ in) tail lift, with 15–19 cm (6–7½ in) nose lift to keep it clear of waves.

Rail Shape
Razor-sharp rails were once high fashion, but are now generally considered obsolete. The usual thing is to compromise between the two extremes of 'hard' (maximum water release for maximum speed) and 'soft' (maximum grip for maximum control) with bevels or chines giving a 'tucked-under' rail that has a clearly defined release edge.

Maximum rail thickness is usually around the mastfoot area, where it overcomes any tendency of the rail to trip or carry straight on when it should be turning.

Bottom Shape
The highly popular double concave gives a trimaran effect which is excellent for marginal planing, but inhibits manoeuvrability more than a pure V or rounded bottom which tends to be found on a wave-orientated short board design.

The bottom shape can be split into three sections, which like the rails must flow smoothly into one another.

Nose section
A flat shape will give maximum lift, but will be very susceptible to chop. Therefore wider nosed boards have this section either slightly veed, rolled or concaved.

Mid section
A flat shape provides optimum lift, but as wind and chop increase it is better to incorporate a fair bit of V with concaves on either side.

Concaves and V in excess of 10 mm (⅜ in) will tend to make the board slower to plane than shallower concaves, but with better control at high speed due to their ability to break up chop. Quad and quinto concaves are useful on wider, lighter wind boards. They provide extra lift.

Tail section
V allows the board to be set deeper in the water, and ensures extra lateral resistance and control over water release. The depth of the V should be compatible with the tail width.

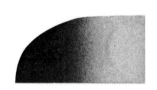

Hard Rail

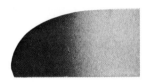

Soft Tucked Rail

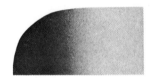

Full Hard Rail

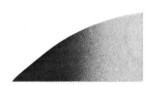

Fine Hard Rail

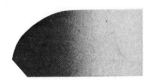

Chined or Bevelled Rail

Volume Distribution of a General Purpose Wave Board

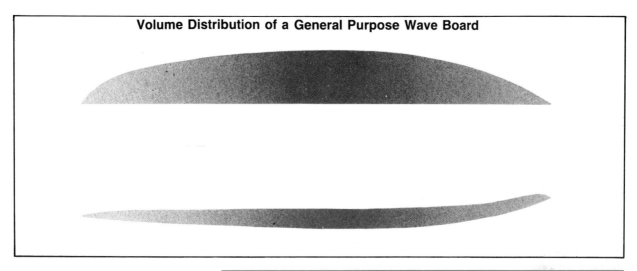

Above: The principal factors which the shaper has to play with include outline and rocker line, rail shape, and volume distribution.

The diagram above shows a typical volume distribution for a wave board which has been designed for use in a wide range of wind conditions. It has maximum volume located near the wide point, tapering to the nose and tail.

Left: Rail shapes alter for different parts of the board's length. Design ranges from low and hard at the tail through full and soft in the middle to low and soft at the nose. Bevels and chines are excellent compromise designs used to smooth out extremes and ensure that it all 'flows'.

Right: Brian Hinde's 'jet bottom' on the Masterclass 295 looks fairly complex, but is no more than a variation on the double concave which works so well with a marginal/fresh wind 295. Note that the rider is sailing with the small thruster fins removed; this is often done to give more speed.

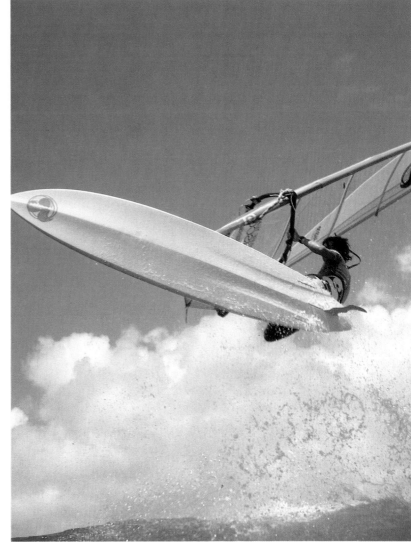

Fins

On a short board the fin is the only thing in touch with the water, which makes it incredibly important if you are going to be able to sail in a straight line and not go sliding off to leeward.

Fin Construction

Most fins are mass produced, being moulded in polycarbonate or glass filled polycarbonate. The second material is stiffer and stronger which is vital for maximum performance.

The strongest of all fins are usually custom made. These fins are cut from sheets of glassfibre and then hand foiled to perfection. Obviously this hand work does mean a much higher price than for a moulded variety of fin.

If you have a custom fin, take care that its leading and trailing edges don't get damaged by running aground. Any ragged edges will seriously impair the fin's performance.

If you are buying a moulded fin, check its stiffness by hand, and in particular check that the base is strong enough to withstand the tremendous sideways pressure that can snap off a bad one in a fast gybe or when landing from a jump. Losing a fin can be very troublesome and even dangerous – the only way you can 'sail' back is in a semi-waterstart position.

Fin Evolution

Early windsurfer fins were all surf style dolphin shapes, and much improved variations on that theme are still popular as shown by the photos on the right. In between times there have been a number of developments designed to make fins both faster and less prone to frequent spin-out.

Fences

Fences are like three or four little wings on the fins. They are there to make the water release cleanly from the trailing edge, rather than flowing straight down from the

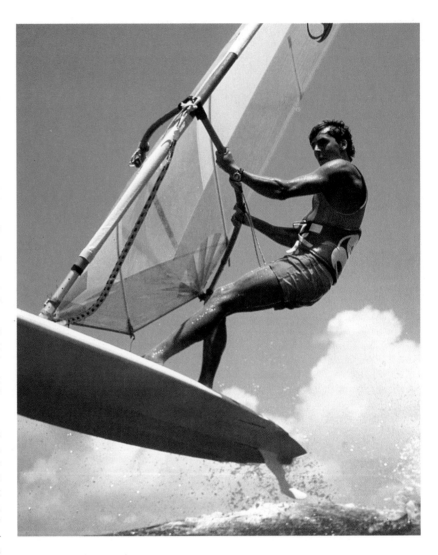

Above: Hopping along with the fin (a Toucan variation) the only thing in contact with the water.

base (where the fin fits into the board) to the tip.

Footballs

Football fins first appeared around 1984, and heralded a new type of design which had a narrow base with a wide tip, designed to make the fin faster (less drag) and prevent spin-out by inhibiting water flow down from the base.

The football was soon replaced by the foot fin which is a football sliced in half, in an attempt to reduce drag problems further. Most recently the cut-out fin (shown right) has appeared. This returns to the old dolphin style with the cut-out in the trailing

edge, making the base much narrower. It has much improved foiling.

Generally speaking, a narrow tail holds in better and only requires a single fin. The less fin area there is the less drag there will be, so this is the general recipe for speed boards.

Wave boards have wide tails if they are for marginal or average wave conditions when flotation is so important. A wide tail will usually have a couple of thrusters.

People get carried away with thrusters, and believe that with a pair of big ones their board will never spin-out or bounce out of a gybe. However if thrusters have too much area the board will plane on the fins when it's going really fast, which will make it flip on its outer rail and bear away of its own volition. The thrusters shown are as big as you'll ever need.

The stiffest combination is thrusters all the way forward and big fin all the way back; moving all the fins back is a typical set-up for choppy water; big fin forward and thrusters back loosens the board, but still maintains enough grip for choppy water.

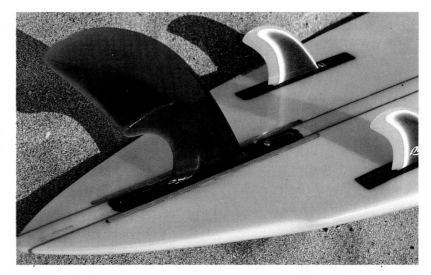

On the asymmetric board shown here, the top turn side of the tail is wide and floaty with a small thruster for extra grip. The bottom turn side is long and gunny, and relies on the single main fin for high-speed grip.

On a board with a conventional outline, a single thruster is sometimes used for extra grip in bottom turns if it is very bouncy and choppy. Basically a thruster or thrusters are needed when extra control is wanted to hold in the rails during high speed gybes.

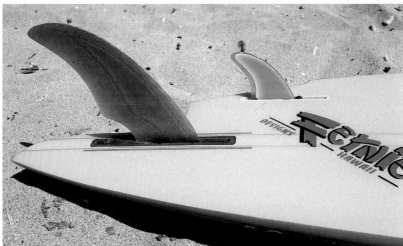

A single fin all the way forward is the loosest possible position. The board is most manoeuvrable and will make the quickest turns, but is also at its most susceptible to spin-out.

With a single fin all the way back the board is still loose, but you have better control during gybes and high speed runs. This is ideal for slalom or the type of speed board shown here with its narrow, gun style tail.

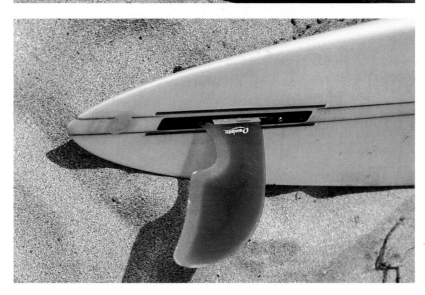

Strap, Fin and Mast Positions

Fin Position

The back of the main box is usually 10–15 cm (4–6 in) from the tail, with the forward thruster boxes level with the front of the main box and as close to the rails as possible. On single fin boards the fin is similarly positioned, with the exception of the all-out speed boards which have the fin as far back as possible.

As a rough guide a tail of less than 27 cm (11 in) – measured 30 cm (12 in) from the tail – will hold in with a single fin, while anything wider needs three fins. For small waves or chop three fins are most suitable; for wide arc turns and high speeds single fins are the norm.

The main fin depth is usually around 22–25 cm (9–10 in), while small thrusters should be no more than half that depth and preferably less. If they are excessive, the board will tend to hydroplane on them during turns and this leads to loss of control.

Mastfoot

The mastfoot is usually around 1.80 m (5 ft 5 in) from the tail. All short boards have some kind of adjustable mastfoot system to allow about 30 cm (12 in) adjustment back or forward.

Start with the mastfoot at eye level with the tail of the board on the ground. If you then put the mastfoot all the way to the back of the box, it will make the board more manoeuvrable since it reduces wetted length by effectively making the board shorter. It can also help jumping, since it assists the board to pivot into the upside-down position more easily.

Good for Speed

Having the mastfoot all the way forward can increase speed. It holds the nose down and stops it bouncing – remember that each

Right: The simplest kind of mastfoot fits into a fin box with a base plate and bolt. Adjustment is easily and quickly accomplished on the beach with a screwdriver, and should not be necessary on the water.

time the nose rises it makes the tail dig into the water. It also makes for a longer, more drawn-out gybe as a result of the increased waterline. However, the board may be more prone to nosediving when jumping.

The shorter the board, the less you need to adjust the mastfoot position. On a 295 the type of sliding track which is adjustable on the water is useful for trimming the board; on anything shorter a simple fin box mastfoot which can be adjusted on the beach is lighter, cheaper and works just as well.

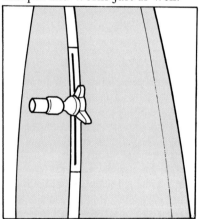

Footstraps

Straps should be spaced to allow a comfortable stance in high winds. A normal stance varies from 50–60 cm (20–25 in), but the positions are to some extent governed by whether the board is being used for speed or wave riding.

It is important that the straps allow the board to ride level for speed, and nose up for turning. 295s have two back straps and sometimes two sets of front straps to allow for this; while shorter boards come down to a simple three strap arrangement.

Always adjust the straps so that your toes peek through but go no further. If your foot slips through during a jump, there could be dire consequences.

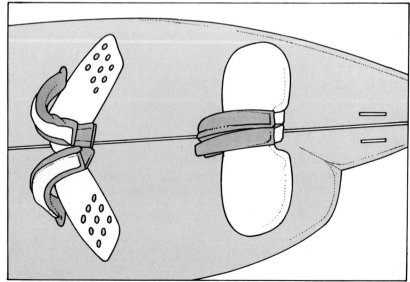

Above: Heavy landings! Thick neoprene pads beneath the footstraps are favoured by sailors who make heavy landings from nine metre (30 ft) jumps. They help prevent dents in the foam.

Harnesses

The harness is used continually for short board sailing – in sub-planing winds of less than 10 knots it's not needed but then you wouldn't be using a short board in these conditions anyway.

Advantages
The human body is not designed for hanging at full arm stretch for long periods of time. So the benefits of using a harness include:
1. More time on the water.
2. Reduced strain on wrists, elbows and shoulders; reduced chance of constricting nerves from overdeveloped wrist muscles.
3. Less damage to palms of hands.
4. Increased rig trim efficiency.

Possible Disadvantages
1. Complete reliance on the harness can be dangerous if it fails.
2. Catapulting when hooked-in can lead to injuries.
3. There is some danger of becoming entangled with harness lines when sailing.

Types
The original waistcoat style of harness provides adequate back support if it is well cut and long enough, and may have good buoyancy which is helpful for learning waterstarts.

However, for short board use the waist or nappy/seat harness is more suitable. This style leaves the top half of the rider's body completely free, and has a lower hook position which allows a more natural unstrained position than the chest high hook on a waistcoat. Whichever style is chosen, the harness needs a spreader bar with at least a 25 cm (10 in) spread.

Harness Lines
Lines should be pre-stretched smooth finish nylon around 15 mm (⅝ in) thick and 96 cm (38 in) long. Most are already sold with webbing/Velcro attachment loops for easy adjustment.

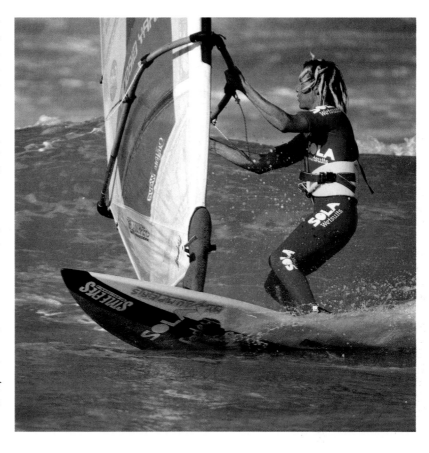

Improperly balanced lines will cause unequal strain on your arms. Also, any change in sail size or wind conditions is likely to mean changing the harness line positions.

Correct balance should be set up on the beach. Hook in to the rig and release pressure on both hands. If the rig falls away from the wind leaving just your back hand on the boom, move the straps forward; if the rig falls into the wind, move the straps back.

You can cover the lines with a plastic tube to make them last longer. Air hose tubing is ideal; you should use two 45 cm (18 in) lengths with an internal diameter to fit the lines. The trouble taken is well worth while: it prevents wear; the lines will never tangle with the hook; the extra weight will making hooking in or out quite easy.

Above: The waist harness allows freedom for the upper body.

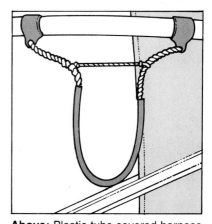

Above: Plastic tube covered harness lines are recommended. The tubing should be centred with 25 cm (10 in) of 3 mm (⅛ in) bungee elastic tied to either side to hold the loop in tension. The lines should be about 35 cm (14 in) apart.

Moulded Board Construction

A short board must be light, but it must also be strong enough to withstand extended use and the stresses which are imposed by sailing in strong wind conditions.

Causes of Damage
Damage may only show up after a couple of years and is likely to take one of the following forms:
1. Impact damage from being dropped on stony beaches, run aground etc. The outer skin may become broken and the foam may be damaged.
2. Delamination of the skin from the foam, or damage to the foam, caused by the pounding of the board by speeding over waves.
3. Complete breakage. In extreme cases a board may be broken in half after a heavy landing.

How Boards are Made
When you're shopping for a short board you'll find a number of options, described here with their advantages and disadvantages.

1. Polyethylene
Advantages: low cost; very durable.
Disadvantages: heavy; very bendy; will not keep its shape.

The simplest form of board construction. The plastic skin is blow or roto moulded, and is very hard wearing. It is filled with polyurethane foam which governs the weight of the board. Polyurethane is fairly heavy, so most polyurethane short boards tend to have low volume.

2. Polyester Glassfibre
Advantages: low cost; quite light and quite stiff.
Disadvantage: not very durable.

A middle of the road construction system which is attractive for small manufacturers since it has low tooling costs. The top and bottom halves of the board are made in glassfibre laminated with polyester resin. The halves are joined around the rails and the board is then filled with polyurethane foam.

Boards using this construction system can be made quite light and stiff, but lightness will be at the expense of durability and quite a lot of care will be needed to keep the board in good condition. The join around the rail will be prone to long term damage.

3. Epoxy Glassfibre
Advantages: very light and very

Below: This cutaway shows a short board with typical composite construction. The core (yellow) is lightweight polystyrene foam, covered with glassfibre rovings and mat (shades of blue) plus carbon fibre reinforcement (red). This is covered with polyurethane resin (pink) before being placed in a heated mould to have the ASA outer skin (white) bonded around it.

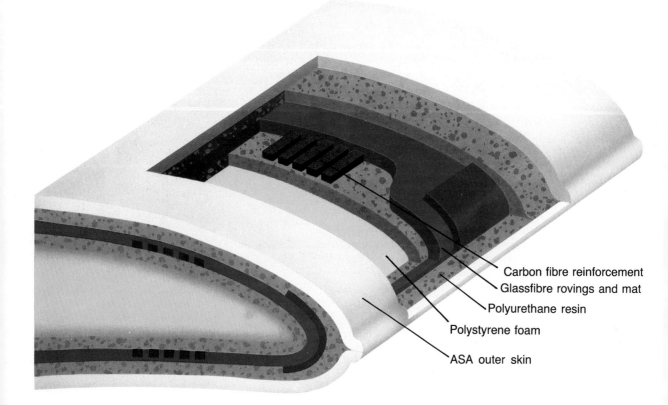

Carbon fibre reinforcement
Glassfibre rovings and mat
Polyurethane resin
Polystyrene foam
ASA outer skin

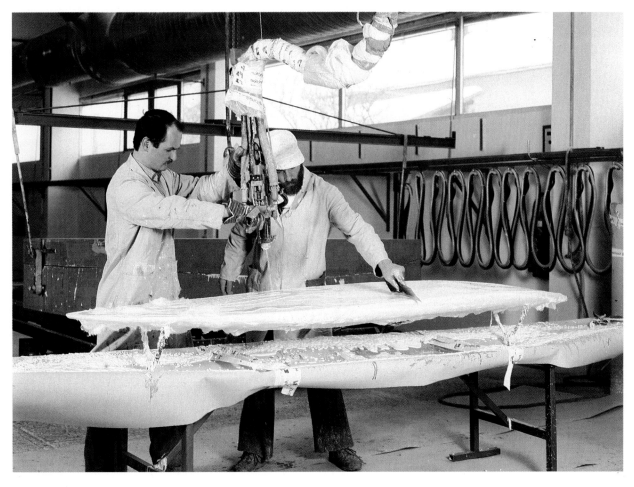

stiff; fairly durable.
Disadvantages: expensive; needs careful looking after.

Epoxy construction makes the lightest and stiffest boards, built round a preformed polystyrene core. This is a much lighter foam (about two-thirds of the weight) than polyurethane.

The glassfibre is laminated with epoxy resin, and the whole lot is baked and compressed in a mould. The resulting board is quite hard wearing, but will still need to be carefully handled. As with most forms of construction, the lighter the board the more fragile it is likely to be.

4. Composite
Advantages: very light and very stiff; quite durable.

Disadvantage: expensive.

Composite boards were pioneered by Mistral with LCS construction. They have a polystyrene core for light weight; an inner glassfibre skin for strength and stiffness; and an outer ASA skin for durability.

This is a complex form of moulded board construction which results in a high price. Composite boards should be almost as stiff and light as epoxy boards, but more durable.

5. ASA/Polyurethane Foam
Advantages: fairly low cost; Disadvantage: quite heavy.

Similar to polyester glassfibre (see left), but also likely to be more durable at the expense of greater weight.

Above: Composite construction. The polystyrene core is wrapped in glassfibre. Polyurethane foam is sprayed all over it, before placing the board in a mould where the ASA skin is bonded round the outside of the board.

6. ASA/Polystyrene Foam
Advantages: fairly low cost; quite light.
Disadvantage: durability.

Polystyrene foam makes the board light, but the great disadvantage is that it does not bond well to the ASA skin which results in long term durability problems, mainly concerned with delamination. The composite form of construction with a layer of glassfibre between the polystyrene and ASA overcomes this problem.

Custom Construction

The world's top board sailors invariably opt for custom boards. There are various reasons why they prefer them to a standard production 'pop out'. These include:
1. A new custom board can incorporate all the latest and up-to-the-minute design details the sailor requires.
2. A custom board is generally very stiff and light, and better in this respect than a production board.
3. A custom board is unique. No other board is quite the same, and even though design may be very similar (many custom boards are made from templates to stock designs) the airbrushed colourwork will ensure that the finished board is a one-off.

The main problem with a custom board is that it is generally quite fragile and will need careful looking after. If you sail from a sandy beach it isn't too difficult to care for your board. But, if you are stuck with pebbles or rock, you will find that the abrasive action of these when the board scrapes aground or is dropped on the shore will inevitably cause damage.

Custom Today – Production Tomorrow

Many successful custom boards become production models, and in fact all the major manufacturers use a 'perfect' specially made custom board as the plug for their moulds. This highly specialized and skilful work has allowed a handful of top shapers to work on a lucrative freelance basis – notably Brian Hinde for Sailboard, Larry McElheny for Fanatic, John Hall for Rainbow (and many others), and the Naish team of Harold Iggey and Rick Naish for Mistral.

Custom Technique

The basics of custom construction have evolved from surfboard design, and the technique is always the same:
The 'shaper' shapes a block of polyurethane or polystyrene foam into the finished board shape.
The 'airbrusher' sprays on the colours and sometimes creates a stunning work of art.
The 'laminator' covers the board with its protective outer skin of glassfibre, using polyester or epoxy resin.

Finally, fittings are bonded into place, and a fantastic high gloss finish is achieved as a result of hours and hours of polishing.

Right: The most famous design team in the world – Rick Naish, son Robby, and their shaper Harold Iggey. Naish Hawaii is based in Kailua, and has designed and made virtually all Robby's competition and wave boards.

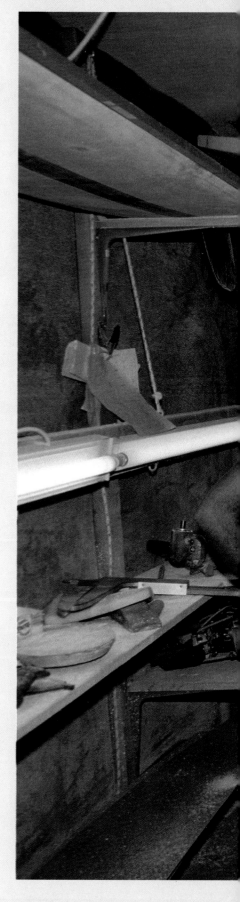

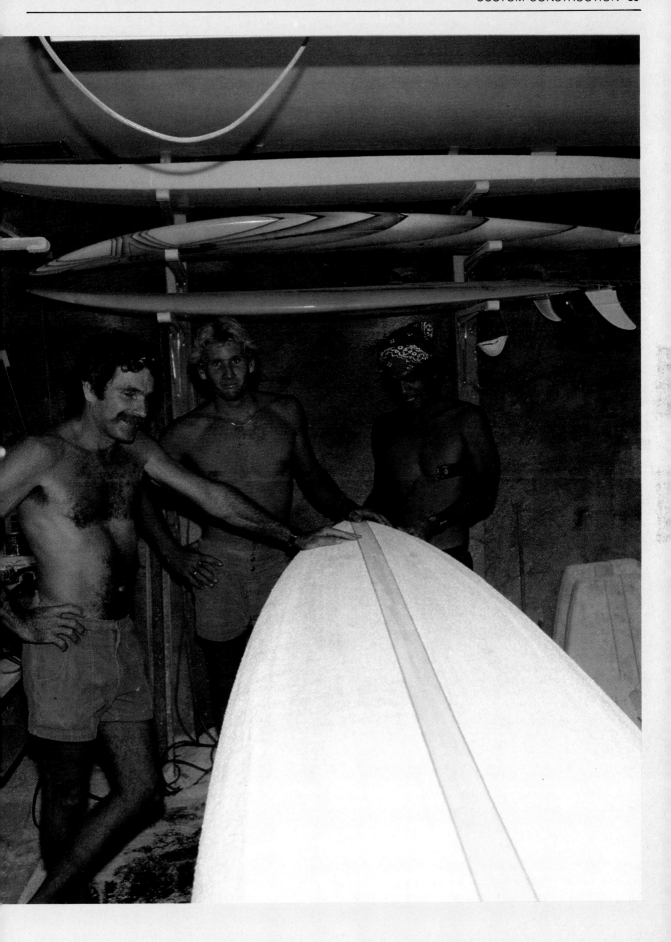

Shaping

The Professionals

Shaping is an art which is achieved only with a great deal of experience. The best professional shapers can turn a foam blank into a finished board shape in under 40 minutes. That time, though, will be considerably lengthened if there are design details such as multi concaves or double wingers.

The professional shaper mainly relies on his eye to make a perfectly symmetrical shape, although he may use fluorescent tubes at the sides of the blank to highlight irregularities. His tools are the saw, manual and electric planes, and varying grades of sandpaper.

The shaper is the lynch-pin in any custom operation. Famous names include Harold Iggey and Jimmy Lewis in Hawaii, and John Hall in the UK. They have star status in the world of performance windsurfing.

Using a Template

It is usually thought that all custom boards are different, but in fact the shapes are often almost identical. Most custom manufacturers will produce a range of 'stock designs', and shape them with the aid of templates taken from the original, which ensures the same performance characteristics.

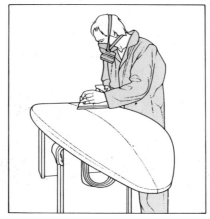

1. Polyurethane foam is the favourite material for the blank with brands such as Clark (USA).

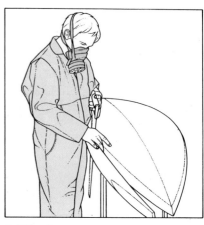

2. The shaper cuts round the plan shape using a saw, before working on the bottom, deck and rails.

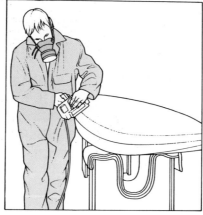

3. Electric planer, hand planer and sandpaper blocks are used for the precise shaping of the rails.

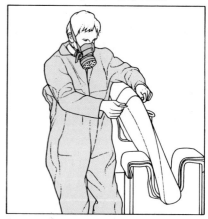

4. When the shape is finished, the blank is sanded with grade 100 paper for a perfect finish.

Airbrushing

The shaped foam is the perfect base for airbrush artistry. Most custom boards have an outer skin which is a laminate of clear resin and glassfibre that becomes as transparent as glass once it has cured. Any designs and colours on the foam can be seen through it, and are protected by the resin during the life of the board, though they fade in strong sunlight.

Airbrushing designs vary from the very basic to extremely complex and artistic work. The longer airbrushing takes, the more you will have to pay. In many cases the skills of a professional artist will be used to paint an 'original' on your board, or copy something such as a picture of Marilyn Monroe.

Painting Technique

Cellulose car paints are used mainly though fluorescent water colours are employed for particularly artistic designs. The technique involves masking the board with tape, spraying the exposed area, and then masking and spraying other areas to build up the desired effect.

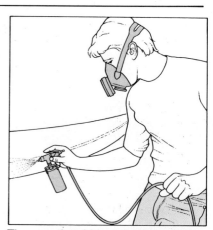

The completed blank is airbrushed with cellulose paint. Masking tape is used to outline the design.

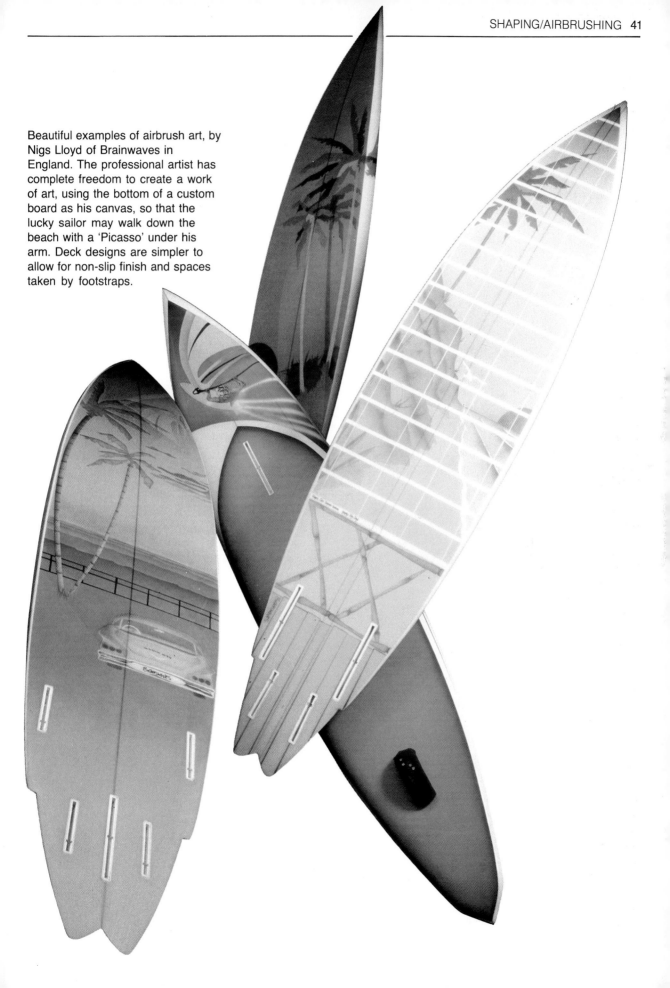

Beautiful examples of airbrush art, by Nigs Lloyd of Brainwaves in England. The professional artist has complete freedom to create a work of art, using the bottom of a custom board as his canvas, so that the lucky sailor may walk down the beach with a 'Picasso' under his arm. Deck designs are simpler to allow for non-slip finish and spaces taken by footstraps.

Laminating

After shaping and airbrushing the custom blank has to be laminated with a glassfibre skin. There are many different types and specifications of glass, but most custom makers favour a woven cloth with two layers on the bottom, and three on the deck plus extra patches around the footstraps, to avoid the danger of heel dents.

The glassfibre is covered with resin – either polyester or epoxy – which 'cures' and turns the soft glass mat into a hard outer skin.

Polyester resin is most widely used since it is easy to work with and relatively cheap. However, it cannot be used together with polystyrene foam since it burns holes in it – hence the need for pricier but stronger epoxy resin.

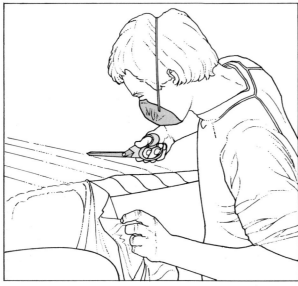

1. The laminator lays the glass cloth on the deck or bottom, and cuts it to the correct shape with an overlap around the rails for good bonding and reinforcement.

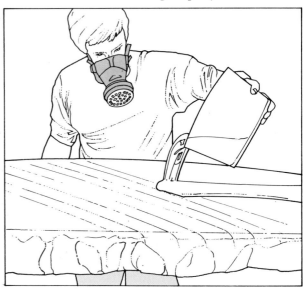

2. The polyester or epoxy resin is poured on to the glass in a carefully measured amount – too little and the glass won't cure correctly, too much and the board is too heavy.

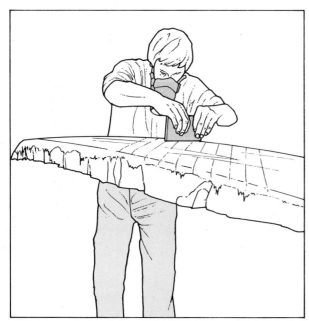

3. A squeegee is used to impregnate the resin, getting rid of any excess and squeezing out air pockets in the laminate. Fast work is imperative before the resin cures.

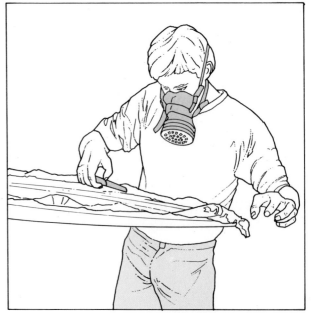

4. A strong overlap at the rails is important since they take all the knocks in use. The resin hardens in about two hours, but it takes at least 24 to be fully cured.

Finishing

A professional custom board maker next puts in the fin box (or boxes), mast track, and footstraps. The usual way is to rout out the correct size holes, and then resin the fittings into position.

Final finishing takes longest of all, and is responsible for the gleaming surface which you see on showroom custom boards. This is the product of three hours or more of power sanding using progressively finer grades of paper, culminating in buffing the board with car polish on a lambswool pad.

Most professionals apply a shiny 'finish coat' composed of resin mixed with wax. Sadly, however, this beautiful finish is virtually impossible to keep after the board has been used a few times.

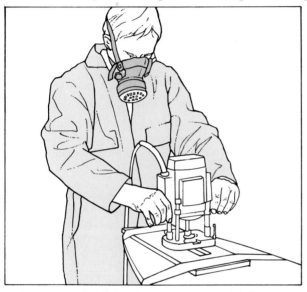

1. Routing out the holes for the fin boxes with a power tool. The polycarbonate/glassfibre boxes are bonded in with glass cloth and resin.

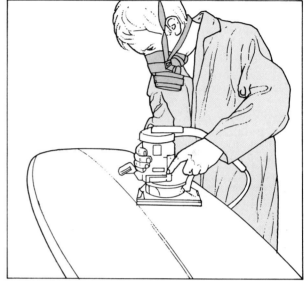

2. Finishing starts with about 90 minutes of light power sanding, after which the shiny finish coat of resin and wax is applied to the top and bottom of the board.

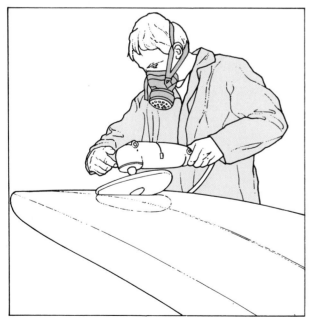

3. Final buffing with a lambswool pad will give the board a fabulous finish which looks great in a shop, but is difficult to maintain after a hard season's sailing.

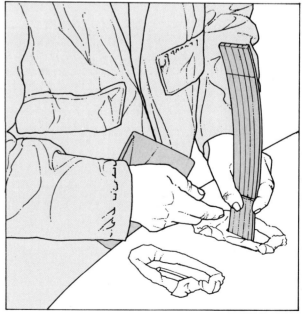

4. Some custom makers fit the footstraps last. Special fittings can be used, but resining the webbing straight into the foam is easiest, quickest, and strongest.

Build Your Own Custom Board

Having read how the professionals do it, you may like to build your own custom board. The example shown on these pages is a 2.50 m (8 ft 2 in) gun which will have about 70 litres volume.

It is primarily designed for flat wave blasting and speed sailing, and with the average weight sailor will require a minimum Force 6 wind to perform well.

The Plan

Each square of the plan represents 2 cm (1 mm = 1 cm scale) and this type of drawing could be used to make any design. Guidelines on construction and a list of tools and materials are given in Appendix III on page 140.

All you need is a workshop or garage; time and patience; money for the materials and tools; great enthusiasm; and a friend who can lend a hand at certain stages. Allow yourself at least six weeks, including weekends.

You could, of course, build a board in polyester and polyurethane, which are the materials most favoured by the professional custom builder. For the amateur, however, epoxy and polystyrene are probably better choices.

Epoxy resin has a longer curing time than polyester resin, which means that you won't have to work so quickly. It can be used with polystyrene or styrofoam which are much lighter and cheaper than polyurethane foam; and it also has a higher strength: weight ratio than polyester.

The three main disadvantages of epoxy are: It is more expensive than polyester resin. It is more difficult to obtain a high quality finish. The board will take a lot longer to construct.

Below: Fancy a speed gun? This is an extreme high wind board developed from competition in international speed weeks.

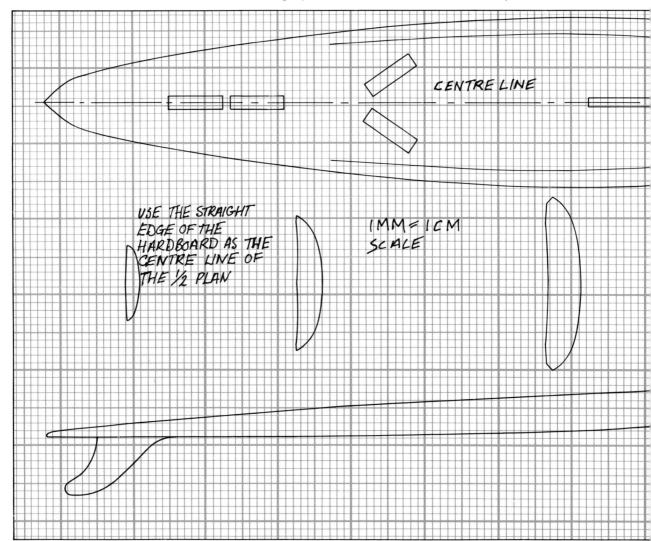

CENTRE LINE

USE THE STRAIGHT EDGE OF THE HARDBOARD AS THE CENTRE LINE OF THE ½ PLAN

1MM = 1CM SCALE

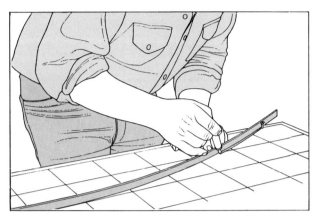

Above: The plan is transferred on to a full scale plan drawn on hardboard. A 'fair curve' (use a batten) is used to draw out the shape by joining dots marked on all the boxes. Templates are then cut out.

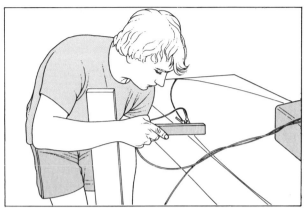

Above: The templates are used to cut the basic shape of the board from the foam, using a home-made 'hot wire'. The length of the hot wire determines the speed of the cut. The next stage will be hand shaping the final shape.

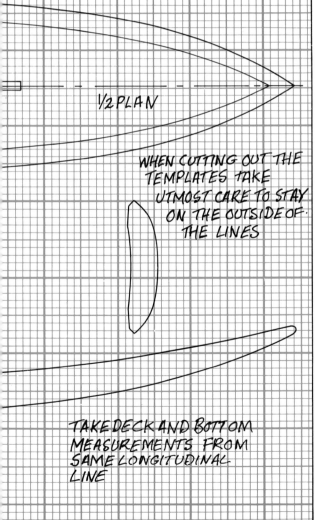

½ PLAN

WHEN CUTTING OUT THE TEMPLATES TAKE UTMOST CARE TO STAY ON THE OUTSIDE OF THE LINES

TAKE DECK AND BOTTOM MEASUREMENTS FROM SAME LONGITUDINAL LINE

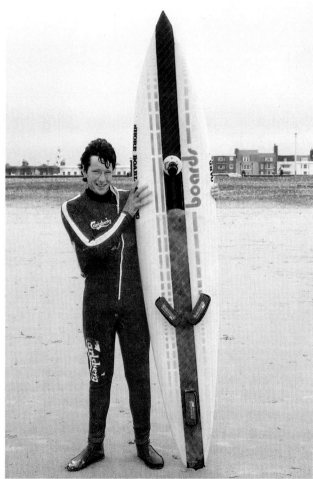

Above: From the plan on the left to the actual board – and it works! This system of amateur construction can be used to create anything from a surfboard to a slalom board.

The Rig

The design of rigs and sails developed at fantastic speed during the early 1980's. Design breakthroughs included the 'Wing' mast (which proved to be a red herring). Other advances, such as tapered battens, rotational cut sails, and camber inducers have helped to make sails more stable, and therefore easier to control in strong winds.

Design changes have been matched by vastly improved materials. Polyester films and polyester woven fabrics are lighter, stronger, and much more stable than old types of sailcloth. Great care still has to be taken, however, to keep them in good condition over two or three seasons.

Types of Rig

Contemporary rigs come in three broad categories. Each has its own advantages and disadvantages.

1. Hard rigs The fully battened, camber induced sail is very stable and very powerful, favoured primarily for speed and control on slalom style 295s, speed boards, and also long World Cup style race boards. The main disadvantages are that the sails are rather heavy, inflexible and ponderous in use.

2. Soft rigs Sails with short battens in the leech (generally with a full length batten in the head, and sometimes the foot) are soft and responsive, but lack the power and drive of the camber induced sail. They are favoured by top wavesailors who demand maximum 'feel' from their sails.

3. Rotationals This is the halfway house between hard and soft, a fully battened rotational sail which always flicks round the mast to set on its leeward side.

The rotation is induced by the battens and the cut and is there to increase both power and control, though in fact few sails will always work perfectly in rotational mode in strong, gusty wind.

Components

The short board sailor requires a mast which is light, fairly stiff, and unlikely to break in the event of a serious wipe-out. The boom should also be light and stiff, as well as fitting perfectly at the mast. Most sailors favour an adjustable boom for use with a number of sails, with a heavy duty adjustable mast extension.

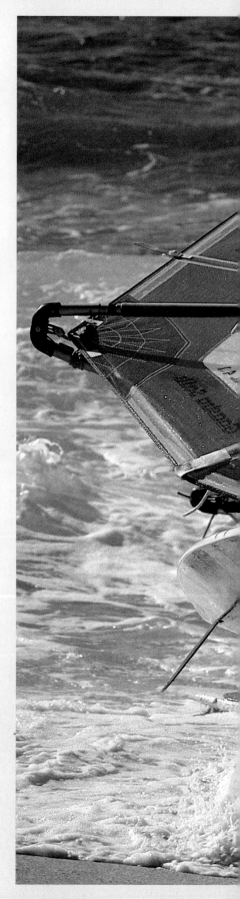

Right: Which is it to be? The DBS (dual batten system, see page 50) or fully battened? The DBS system offers the choice of sailing in the soft mode, or the sail can be rigged as a fully battened rotational or non rotational.

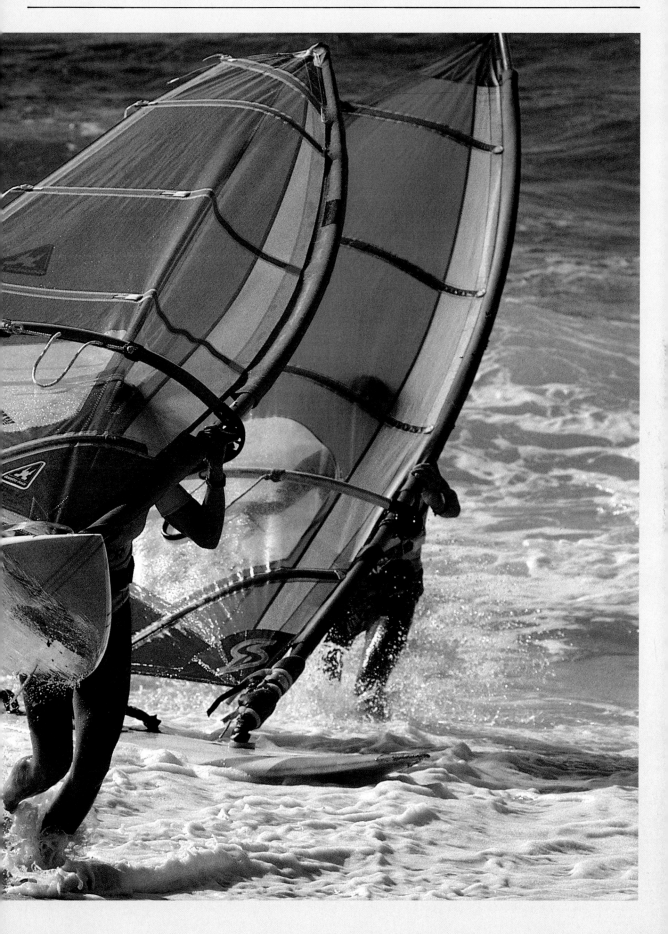

Hi-performance Rigs

The Racer
The racer wants to get there fast! He may be competing in short board slalom or speed trials. In both events the prime requirements are for maximum speed and tight turns.

Designing for Speed
The sail designer creates a fast sail by encouraging airflow to stick to the leeward side of the sail. The pressure difference between the leeward (low pressure) and windward (high pressure) sides must be maintained or the sail cannot keep up maximum speed.

The designer's first step is to minimize wind interference from the mast. This is why rotational and camber induced sails are faster than conventional soft or fully battened types. However, where a camber induced sail really scores is in its engineering and structure, which has the inboard end of the batten so positively attached to the mast that the sail can hold its shape in higher winds better than any other kind of design.

Speed Factors
Whether a racer's sail is camber induced or rotational, there are a number of important points that will add to its speed, and are common to sails of this type used for slalom or speed trials.

1. Luff System
This must be aerodynamically efficient with minute attention to detail – for example fairing in the boom cut-out, and not using a wind-resisting thick uphaul or mast protector pad.

2. Aspect Ratio
Low aspect sails have longer booms which makes them easier to sheet to the correct angle, and will make them faster than an incorrectly sheeted high aspect ratio sail on a broad reach.

On reaches closer than 120 degrees the high aspect sail is comparatively easy to sheet correctly, and with its short

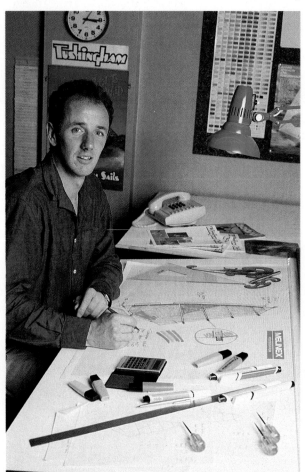

Above: The sail designer at his drawing board. This is Roger Tushingham who produces the best selling range of Tushingham short board sails.

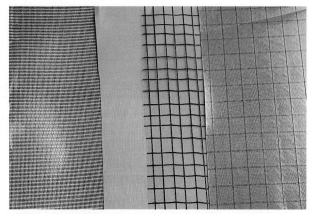

Above: The lightest, most stable materials for high performance short board sails are made from polyester film laminates of the types shown here.

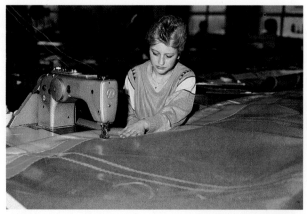

Above: The cutting of a hi tech sail must be very precise as any variation may ruin its sets and performance. This kind of sail construction is labour intensive and costly.

boomed, easy handling characteristics it will be a fast option. As most racing has more close reaching than broad reaching, the high aspect sail is therefore likely to be the better choice.

3. Low Cut Foot

If air is allowed to escape under the foot it will reduce the sail's power. In order to minimize this a racing sail should be cut as low as possible to close the gap between board and sail. This is particularly important in the forward half of the sail where laminar flow is most effective.

4. Sail Twist

The wind has considerably more speed at the top of the mast than at the bottom, where surface friction from the water slows it. The result is that the apparent wind direction (the combination of the true wind and the wind caused by the board's speed) is close to the centreline of the board lower down in the sail. Therefore the sail must be able to twist open towards the top if it is to have the correct angle of attack along its length.

To achieve the right kind of twist a high aspect ratio racing sail needs a lot of area built into the head, so the leech below it is almost straight down.

This outline shape will encourage an even twist with the leech most open at the top. If more area is added to the leech it will tend to twist open too low down with a resulting loss of efficiency.

Summary

A fast sail incorporates a combination of factors which should give the following: speed in a straight line; stability in strong winds; and also allow adequate manoeuvrability for gybing.

The Wave Sailor

The wave sailor also needs a high performance sail, but this doesn't

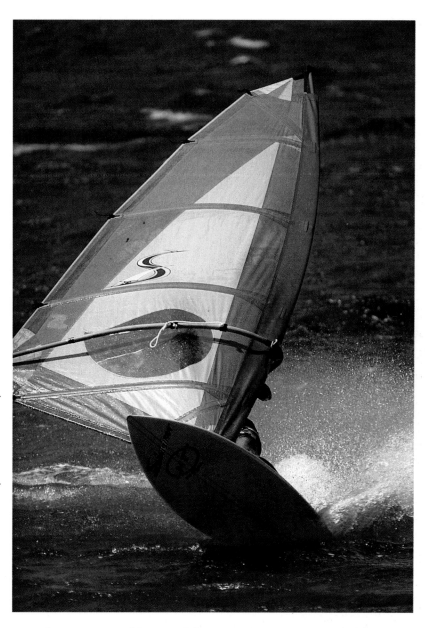

mean he wants speed in a straight line. He is looking for fast action on the wave face with lightning manoeuvres and big jumps. He also wants a sail that will stay in one piece!

1. Outline

A wave sail should be reasonably high aspect for allround performance and easy handling. Never go for extremes – a super high aspect sail will be very twitchy with poor

Above: The camber induced sail combines stability and power for slalom racing but is comparatively clumsy for recreational use.

offwind performance; super low aspect will be too cumbersome and slow for manoeuvres.

Manoeuvrability is the major influence on the outline of a wave sail. The clew must be cut high enough to prevent it from catching on the water, and the foot must be cut so the sailor has no problem with radical manoeuvres such as duck gybes and 360s, with only a small amount of extra foot area built in near the tack to put more power in the sail.

The trailing edge of the sail will need to be built out at the head to promote the right amount of twist, as on a racing sail. The big difference is that in waves the top half of the sail is often much more important than the bottom half.

2. Luff System

Camber inducers are no use to a wave sailor. What is needed is a tightly cut luff tube which won't fill with water, so that the sailor can make quick recoveries from falls; and the lightest sail tends to be the most manoeuvrable.

Sometimes a wave sailor will need maximum power from the sail, at other times he will find there is too much power to handle. The sailmakers have to some extent come up with an answer to this with the Dual Batten System, or DBS, which is featured widely on wave sails.

The idea is simple enough. The two battens directly above the boom can either be short or full length, so that the sail can be adjusted from fully rotational through to soft by using the correct battens with the outhaul and downhaul controls.

Therefore the sailor can opt for the most rigid rotational flowshape to give maximum aerodynamic efficiency in variable conditions when he needs power to get out through the waves.

In more stable, big wave conditions he can pull hard on the outhaul and downhaul which will transform the sail into a fully battened non rotational, with the long battens stabilizing the flowshape as he goes through high speed manoeuvres on the wave face, but without the power locked in as it is with a rotational.

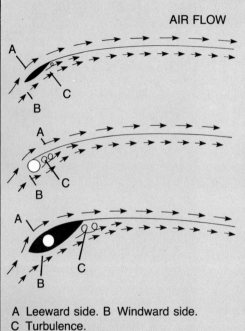

AIR FLOW

A Leeward side. B Windward side.
C Turbulence.

A sail is driven by airflow along the windward and leeward sides. The slow moving air on the windward side creates high pressure; the fast moving air on the leeward side creates low pressure. It is the pressure difference between the two which drives the sail.

These three diagrams – wing (top), rotational (centre), and foam wing (bottom) – show how sailmakers have tried to create smooth flow along both sides with minimum turbulence behind the mast.

LIFT

A sail should drive you forwards if your priorities are speed and power. A non rotational sail with an even camber generates its lift sideways (right); a camber induced or rotational sail generates most of its lift into direct forward power (left).

Changing the long battens for short ones makes the sail soft, so that it can be partially depowered during tight manoeuvres without affecting control – a mode that is ideal for small waves.

Overall the dual batten system gives maximum flexibility to one sail, which is a most useful feature for the serious wave sailor.

3. Window

Wave sailors appreciate a big window, extended upwards for viewing the top of the wave during bottom turns and downwards for

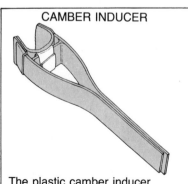

CAMBER INDUCER

The plastic camber inducer joins the full length batten directly to the mast.

allround visibility off the lip.

Apart from being able to see what the wave is doing, it is important to be able to check what other sailors are up to – in this respect it's also a lot safer to have a brightly coloured sail. It is always best to see and be seen!

4. Construction
Wave sails are obviously used in extreme conditions and need to be super strong to withstand the incredible forces in play when you have fallen in a wave break. You will also find a handle at the mast head a useful extra – it's a good way to keep a handhold.

Summary
The wave sailor's ideal sail is quite different from the racer's, even though both have emerged as a result of applying simple common sense to problems encountered.

The Recreational Sailor
Most sailors fall into this category. You may do the odd race and sometimes sail seriously in waves, but few sailors do it often enough to justify specialist equipment.

Racing and wave sails have numerous drawbacks which make them unsuitable for allround fun. The recreational sail compromises on the best points of both race and wave sails in order to have good speed and good manoeuvrability, even though it will not be the ultimate in either department.

When looking at the features of a recreational sail you should ask yourself: *Do I need this feature? What are its advantages? Are there any disadvantages?*

1. Luff System
This is where you must decide on induced, rotational, or soft.

Right: Maximum area at the head so that the sail twists off correctly; maximum area in the foot to close up the slot for the racer.

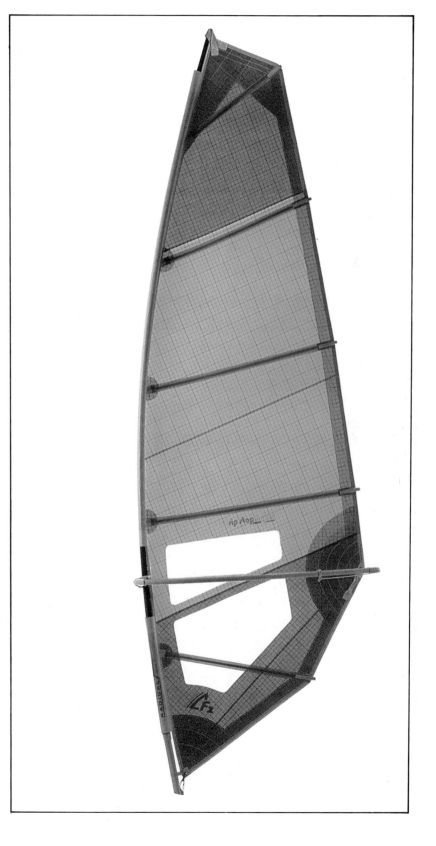

If you are interested in speed you must go for the first two and add up their plus and minus points. In fact for recreational use the rotational sail has many more pluses – it's lighter, easier to rig, safer (the luff will not fill with water), cheaper, and almost as aerodynamically efficient.

In comparison the camber induced sail has a slight speed edge combined with more stable handling in a straight line.

2. Outline
It is easy to combine the best points of a racing and wave sail to make a good compromise outline for a recreational sail.

The trailing edge should have most of the sail area concentrated near the top to create the right twist characteristics. At the foot of the sail there should be enough area for power and closing the slot, but not so much that you're unable to perform duck gybes and easy manoeuvres.

3. Window
A reasonably sized window which gives a wide view will make life easier for the recreational sailor.

Summary
Avoid anything extreme. Radical features which produce a few advantages will almost certainly

have equally significant drawbacks. A good recreational sail should be a mellow combination of proven features which will produce a good allround result, with as much as 90 per cent of the specialist sail's advantages and none of its disadvantages.

Modern Materials
The proliferating number of brands and trade names make materials used in sail making seem confusing. They can, however, be

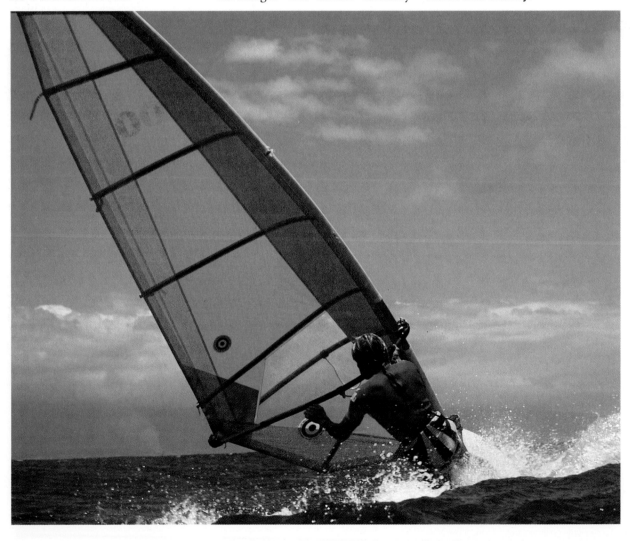

Below: Going for a gybe with a full length (tapered) batten sail and woven fabric and film sail providing almost total stability.

broken down into three basic forms:

1. ***Woven fabric.***
2. ***Film.***
3. ***Woven fabric and film laminate.***

There are four basic materials:

1. ***Nylon.***
2. ***Polyester.***
3. ***PVC.***
4. ***Aramatic polymides.***

Almost all the hi tech sail fabrics fit within these groups, and a glossary of the most popular brand names and generic terms is given in the appendix on page 142.

Material Development

In the early days windsurfing sails were cheap and cheerful but very poor performers. They were made out of loosely woven polyester fabrics with cheap resin finishes which gave initial stability, but soon broke down into soft, baggy and inefficient sails.

Sailmakers then began to use more tightly woven polyester fabrics with much harder resin finishes, and this material would last much longer. However it was quite heavy, and with the availability of polyester films (Mylar etc) the practice of laminating film on to lightweight woven fabric was introduced.

The low stretch of the film and the strength of the fabric combined to give much lighter cloth with as good if not better performance.

This type of cloth is still widely used, but from being a one-sided laminate has developed into a 'three ply' laminate with two layers of film sandwiching the woven fabric. In many cases this woven fabric has become a fairly loose 'scrim' of robust yarn with an easily recognizable criss-cross pattern inside the see-through film material, as shown in the photograph on page 48. The film provides stability, while the scrim is tear resistant, and makes the sail reasonably easy to sew.

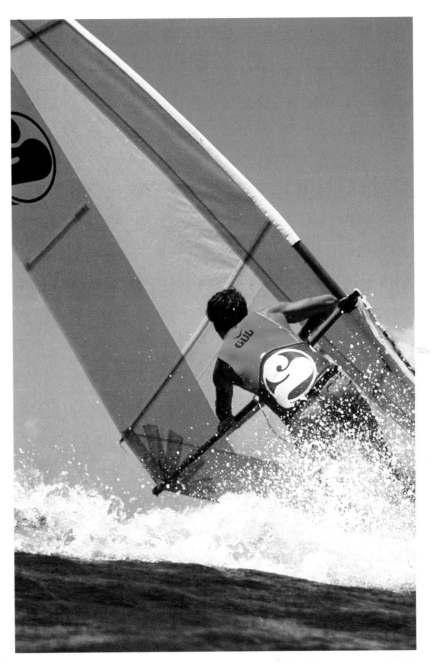

Typical materials used are:
Main body: Lightweight tri laminate material.
Luff tube: Heavy duty nylon.
Luff, leech, foot: Hard resin finished woven polyester.
Clew, tack, head panels: Hard resin finished woven polyester forming tapered corner patches.
Window: PVC or polyester film.

Above: The 'soft' sail has two short battens in the leech above the boom, making the sail more responsive and easier to depower, but less stable for straight line blasting.

DBS sails have a double batten pocket which allows you the option of sailing with full length or short battens to suit your sailing style and the conditions.

Setting the Rig

Modern high performance rigs are easy to set, and you should be able to make them wrinkle free with the right power characteristics for use on the water. Whichever mode, the rigging and derigging sequence will follow the same pattern, with small variations for soft, fully battened, and camber induced sails. The sequence below assumes you have a brand new sail.

Rigging Sequence

1. Take it out of the bag, unroll it, and lay it flat on the ground. If possible make sure that your rigging area has a non abrasive surface. Concrete in particular is notorious for damaging sails, rubbing away the fragile polyester film of sailcloth.
2. Slide the mast up the luff tube. If it's a tight fit, it may go up more easily when wet. Slide it right through to the head.
3. Fit the mastfoot. It is unlikely that your sail will

match exactly the length of your mast. You will need an adjustable mast extension, adjusted so that the tack of the sail comes as low down as possible. Put on light downhaul tension.
4. Work out where you want the boom on the mast. Between chin (waveriding) and nose (slalom) is about right for most short board users. The easiest way to do this is to measure up the boom against your body, and then lay it along the mast.
5. Attach the boom using whichever inhaul method is suitable for a tight fit. The Hawaiian inhaul shown overleaf is the most basic. Don't make it too tight, or you may crush the mast.
6. Straighten out the boom, taking great care to keep it straight so that the jaws pass each side of the mast. Make up the outhaul and tension it.
7. Slide in the full length battens, and tension each one very carefully.

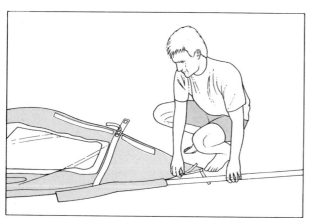

1. Slide the mast up the tube. If you have inducers, make sure the mast passes up through them correctly. Full length battens may need slackening a few inches.

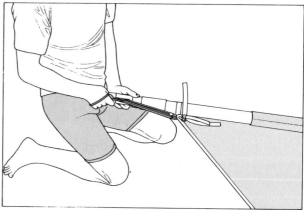

2. Push in the mastfoot. Unless mast and sail are perfectly matched for length, you will need an adjustable extension to get the sail down near to the deck.

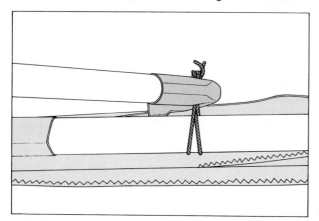

5. Don't overtighten the inhaul or you may crack the mast when you straighten out the boom. Take great care to keep the cheeks aligned on either side.

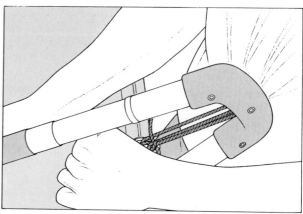

6. Straighten the boom, and make up the inhaul. If the sail is camber induced or rotational it is likely to need very little tension – pulling too tight spoils the shape.

8. Lastly, fine tune the battens, outhaul and down-haul to get the set you require.

Variations in Settings

Soft sails: On some soft sails you can only put in the short battens when the sail is untensioned; in other words before you outhaul the boom.

Fully battened sails: If the battens are already in the sail, you may have difficulty straightening out the boom due to the amount of camber in the bottom battens. You may need to take out the bottom battens so you can pull the boom round to fix the outhaul. Then replace the battens.

Camber inducers: These are fiddly! There are little pockets in the luff tube so you can wriggle them into position before inserting the mast. Make sure the mast passes up cleanly through them.

Dual batten systems: You will always need to ease

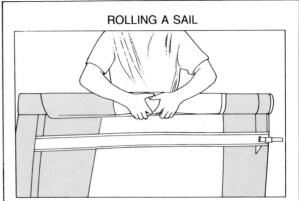

ROLLING A SAIL

Above: The easiest way to put away a sail is to roll it around the battens. You may need to pull out the bottom ones. Release tension on them all.

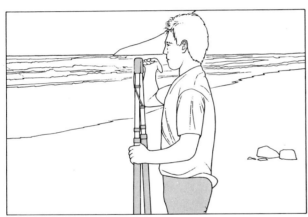

3. Having applied light downhaul tension, work out where you want the boom height, and if you use a regular sail, mark it with a piece of tape.

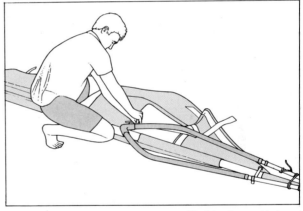

4. Lay the boom along the mast, with the clew end down by the foot. Most booms have very efficient inhaul systems which lock the boom tightly.

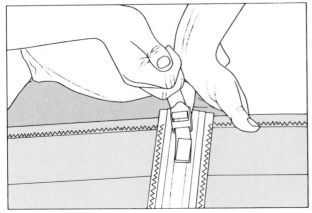

7. Slide home the full length battens, making sure they fit correctly into the luff. Adjust the buckles for tension – this should remove all wrinkles along the pockets.

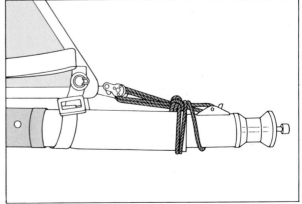

8. Finally tune the outhaul, battens, and downhaul and tie them off securely. The tack should be pulled in close to the mastfoot, as shown, by using the webbing strap.

both outhaul and downhaul to make the fully battened sail rotational. Tightening outhaul and downhaul will make the sail non rotational.

Correct Set

A fully battened sail virtually holds its own shape and is very easy to set. If it is rotational or camber induced too much outhaul or downhaul will simply make it less effective. However if you feel there is too much wind for the sail you can flatten it by tightening the outhaul. This will cut down the power and make it easier to handle.

Because of its less rigid frame, a soft sail can be difficult to set. Here are some common problems:

Is the mast right for the sail? Some bend too much, some too little. Ask your retailer or sailmaker whether your mast is suitable.

Is the boom right? It must have the correct angle at the jaws to accommodate the camber in the sail. It must also be stiff enough not to flex and distort the shape of the sail in a gust.

Vertical creases? Try less downhaul or more outhaul.

Horizontal creases? Try less outhaul or more downhaul.

Batten creases? Put more tension on the battens.

Putting the Sail Away

It's a good idea to hose off any salt water with fresh water. Salt is very abrasive and will damage the sail-cloth in time.

Always ease off the downhaul before letting off the outhaul. This prevents overloading the luff. Let off tension on all the battens, and if necessary remove the bottom ones to take off the boom.

Roll the sail from head to foot and then put it away in its bag. This is the best way to store your sail.

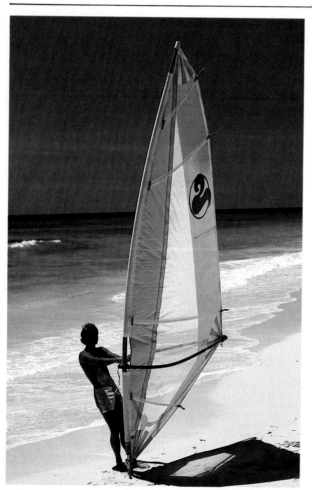

If the mast is the right stiffness and the boom the right stiffness and shape, all you need is to adjust outhaul, downhaul and batten tension to shape the sail.

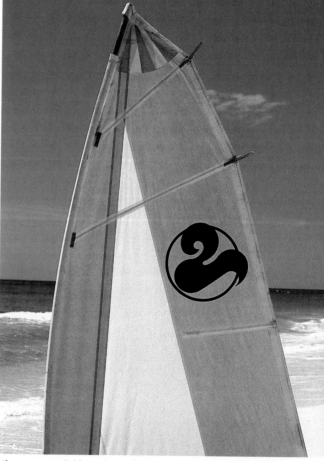

If there are crinkles along the batten pockets, tighten the battens until they disappear. Take note that the pockets are very vulnerable to abrasion on dry land when rigging.

FITTING A CAMBER INDUCER

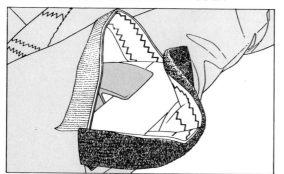

Camber inducers usually have little pockets in the luff tube fastened by Velcro or a zipper. After fiddling them in, you can leave them in position.

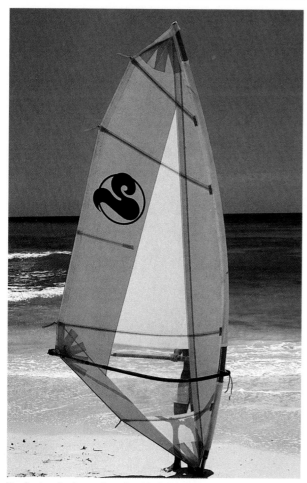

Perfect set of a soft sail with fully battened head and short battens in the leech. The boom should be horizontal, and between chin and nose when you're sailing.

HAWAIIAN INHAUL

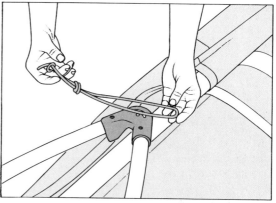

1. The Hawaiian inhaul is a basic system for getting a tight fit which always works. Start by doubling a short line, then tie an overhand knot.

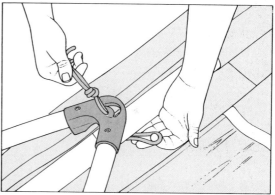

2. Slip the loop end through the hole in the boom, and round the back of the mast. You can then pass it over the knot, which locks it into position.

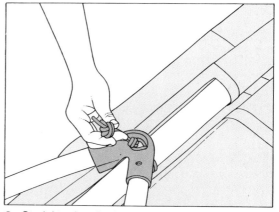

3. Straightening the boom will give you a rock hard inhaul fitting, but the knot must be in exactly the right place. Trial and error is the only method.

Basic Technique

This section covers all the techniques which will be needed by those who are new to short board sailing. To master them in safety the best board is a 295 with around 120 litres volume. This will have the responsiveness and speed for you to enjoy everything that is best about short board sailing. It will also have sufficient flotation and size to keep you out of trouble, by allowing uphauling if you can't waterstart, and carrying you through gybes which would stall a small board.

Starting out Safely

Unless you are very light don't make the mistake of buying a short board which is too small. It may be comparatively easy to sail and fast in a straight line, but you should not sail one until you're 100 per cent proficient at carve gybes and waterstarts on a longer board. Firstly, you're going to be in real danger if you suddenly find you can't waterstart, and secondly, a low volume board will stall and sink so readily that it will be extremely hard for you to make any progress in learning gybing technique.

Best Conditions for Learners

Most short board sailors like nothing better than blasting out on a beam reach, gybing without falling off (which wastes time and lets you drift downwind); then reaching back in, and gybing once again to repeat the process. If there are waves you should be able to jump the board fairly easily on the way out, riding back in on the waves.

To do all this, you will need good sideshore conditions – either blowing from left to right or right to left. Side on or side offshore can be almost as good, but full offshore or onshore are to be avoided, as is high water where there's a steep shelving shoreline which will promote waves that make launching difficult or impossible.

So read on and find out how you can reach out, do a few jumps, carve a smooth gybe, ride waves on the way back in, throw a fast gybe on the inside, and carry on all day – or at least until you're satisfied and exhausted.

Right: Bearing off to carve gybe a short board of around 2.65 m (8 ft 8 in), this is World Champion Robby Naish at his favourite sailing location – Diamond Head, Oahu, Hawaii.

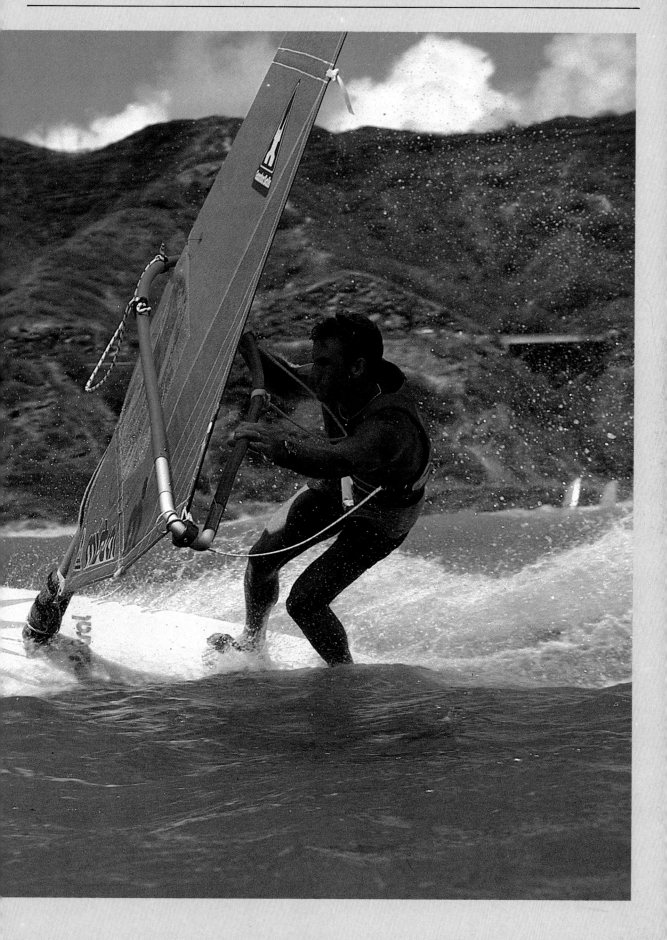

Carrying Board and Rig

A short board is unlikely to weigh more than 12 kg (26 lbs), and with low volume may be little more than half that. The rig may add another eight kg (18 lbs), so with a total of 20 kg (44 lbs) the complete unit still weighs less than many long boards.

If you use the wind to help lift the rig, it is fairly easy to carry both board and rig a short way down to the water. Always keep to the same carrying sequence when moving your gear.

The Carrying Sequence
1. Lie the board on the beach, and point it in the direction you wish to go – presumably out to sea!
2. Fix the mastfoot securely, and place the rig the right way round for sailing, with the mast to windward, and the boom end lying downwind.

Right: Technique is more important than strength when carrying a short board and rig together. Use the wind to help you – don't fight it.

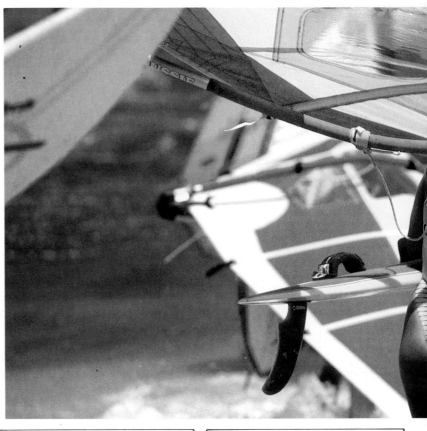

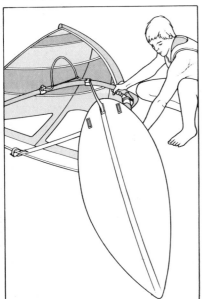

1. This technique is used for carrying longer distances, when the conventional method is too tiring. Align board and rig with the nose upwind and the mast tip downwind.

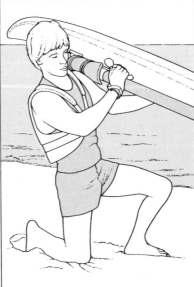

2. Kneel down so you can lift the board on to your shoulder. Face the tail if the wind is offshore (behind you) or the nose if it's onshore (towards you). Stand up.

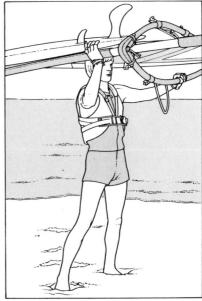

3. The sailor supports the board with one hand, and the boom with the other. (Face the opposite way for onshore winds.) You can walk a surprising distance like this.

Short Board Launch

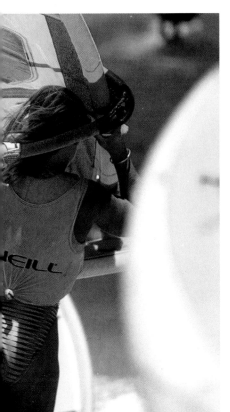

Conditions for launching will be dictated by the launch area, the state of the tide (if any), and the wind. If the water is flat and there are no rocks it is relatively easy.

Onshore Winds
Winds that are side-onshore pile up the waves and make it difficult to get away from the beach. The more onshore the wind, the more problems you will have. Carry the board in as deep as possible and wait for a gap in the waves before dropping it on the water and stepping on. Even the smallest waves have a surprising amount of power which will sweep you shorewards (and usually off the board) if you

don't have enough speed when you hit them.

Offshore Winds
There are unlikely to be waves, unless they are the remainder of earlier wind conditions. Your problem will be a flukey wind which gets stronger as you go further offshore.

Dumpers
Dumpers are waves which build up and crash down on a steeply shelving beach, usually at high tide. They have immense power which can break masts and even boards. There may also be a dangerous undertow.

3. Grab the mast with your front hand, just below the boom. Grab the nearside front strap with your other hand.
4. Lift the mast to shoulder height. If the wind is sideshore, this will be very easy.
5. Stick your head beneath the boom so you're looking through the window in the sail, and then stand up straight, lifting both board and rig. You can now walk down the beach and can use the same procedure on the return.

Strong or Gusty Winds
To maintain control in strong and gusty winds is quite a knack. Always make sure that the boom is pointing the same way as the wind, and adjust the board to an angle where all its weight is being carried by the rig. This may be flat (see main picture) or with the nose of the board pointing upwards.

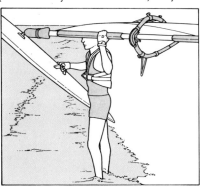

1. Carrying board and rig in classic style, with the wind blowing from left to right. Holding the nose up unweights the board, but makes it tricky to handle in strong wind.

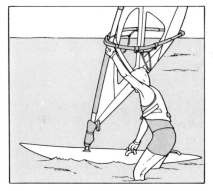

2. Wait for a gap between the waves. Walk in (run if they are dumpers) and drop the board when it's deep enough to clear the skeg with your weight on the tail. Steady the rig.

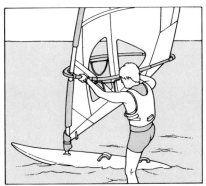

3. Hop up back foot first, but direct all your weight on to the mastfoot so the board won't sink and can accelerate quickly. You must be fast if the board is a sinker.

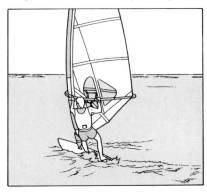

4. Power on and sail off. Frequently it's not so easy – the board sinks or isn't moving fast enough to make it through the first wave. Be ready for a waterstart to get you off again.

Reaching Out and Reaching In

Sailors who live in non tidal areas are likely to have fairly constant and predictable conditions which should make their sailing fairly easy. Those who live in tidal areas will find that conditions will change throughout the day according to the state of the tide.

Problems with Tidal Beaches

Tidal beaches often shelve steeply and then flatten off. This means that at low water the waves are small, easily handled, and ideal for speedsailing; but perhaps disappointing for wavesailing.

At high tide the waves will heap up and break on the steep shore. This can make getting off the beach very difficult and dangerous. Even when you're up on the board the waves may be too closely spaced to allow you to accelerate and build up speed before another wave hits you and stops the board

dead. If the wind is slightly onshore it will also carry you back to the shore.

Using the Half-Tide

The best conditions in a tidal area are often found at half-tide, when you benefit from a compromise between flat water and waves. You can only find out the best state of the tide for an area from your own experience – or by watching and enquiring locally.

Reaching Out

A wind that is sideshore with a tolerance of about 45 degrees on either side should present few problems. You can sail at near full speed away from the shore, and head the board directly into oncoming waves.

Close in, these waves are likely to be breaking, and when you hit an oncoming wall of white water

it will immediately stop the board and throw you forward.

Overcoming Waves

To counteract hitting waves you have to lift the nose, pushing your weight on to the back foot and absorbing the sudden lift of the board with your legs.

The board will be slowed, so if necessary pump the rig to bring it back on to the plane. If there is a space between the waves, choose the unbroken sections to sail over.

The closer you get to the breaking section, the steeper the wave will be. This makes it the best part for jumping (see page 70) but the worst place possible for keeping up speed.

Below: Reaching out in a side offshore wind. The leeward rail will hit the oncoming waves first, so you must lean back and lift the rail.

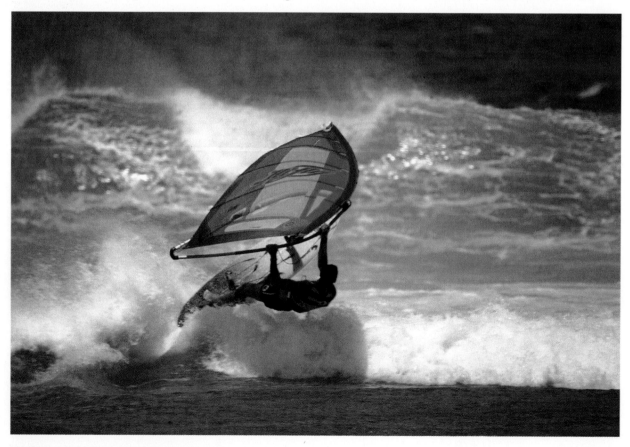

Getting Out in Offshore Winds

Sailing out in offshore winds is fast and easy on a broad reach. Waves will be small since they are flattened by the wind.

If you sail out on a close reach in an offshore wind the leeward rail will hit the wave first. You should therefore push down on the windward rail to lift the leeward side, and at the same time lean back against the rig to pull against the increased force in the sail.

Reaching In

Once clear of the shorebreak you can reach out over clearer water before gybing, and then reach back in. In sideshore and side-onshore conditions this is likely to be a fast trip, as you can ride and surf the waves all the way back.

In offshore winds you will have to compromise between riding waves and the need to keep heading high to return to your start point.

In onshore winds your speed on the waves will substantially reduce the apparent wind in the sail, so you rely more on surfing than windsurfing techniques, while correctly weighting and footsteering the board to keep it well under control.

Using the Wave Face

The secret of a high speed ride back to the shore is to keep on a wave face. When you catch the wave bear off to get up speed. You will accelerate rapidly as you take off down the steep face, but, before you outpace it, luff the board and sail diagonally across the wave, using its power to carry you all the way in. As you near the shore gybe out and over the wave before it starts to break up.

Keeping Away from the Beach

If the wind is closer to onshore, you can have problems getting away and staying away from the beach. Oncoming waves will

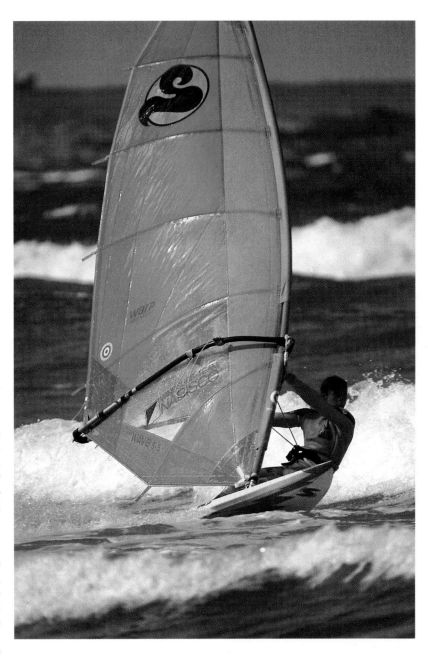

strike the full length of the windward rail and drive you shorewards, depowering the rig and letting you down into the water. You may have to wait for the white water to pass over your head before making a quick waterstart.

The other problem is that your speed will be relatively slow due to your closehauled course, but all you can do is watch for the

Above: Reaching back in becomes a real high speed ride if there are waves and it's a sideshore wind. Bear off to accelerate down the wave, and then head up to stay on its face for as long as possible.

oncoming waves and luff the board up and over them, lifting on the windward rail at the same time to take you cleanly over.

Waterstarts

If you can't waterstart, you can't sail a short board. Apart from the inconvenience, it is often impossible to uphaul a 295 if the wind is strong. Therefore it's essential to master the art of waterstarting before you venture away from the shore on a short board.

The best place to learn is on flat water with a steady Force 3–4 breeze. It helps if you can stand on the bottom, but if not you may find it easier to wear a high buoyancy harness – then at least you don't have to worry about keeping yourself afloat.

Positioning the Rig

When you fall in, the rig is seldom the right way round or on the right side for a quick waterstart. You will have to flip the clew or swim the rig round to get it into the right beam-on position. The nose of the board should point into the wind with the mast at right angles.

The most important thing to remember is that you must keep on swimming the rig forward into the wind, because it will be blown back constantly.

While you're doing this, a sharp tug on the mast just above the boom should be enough to get wind under the sail and free the boom end from the water.

While you're learning the waterstart, the best way to swim may be to try a sort of backstroke into the wind, while pushing the mast up with your hands.

Once the boom end comes free

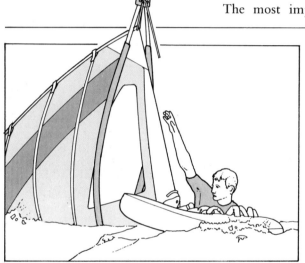

1. Rig the wrong way round and on the wrong side. First lift the boom end until the wind gets under it. You can then flip it so that it's the right way round.

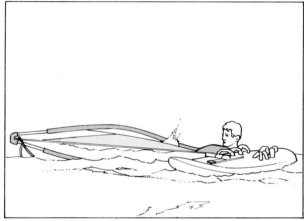

2. With the mast upwind, swim the rig into the wind round the tail of the board until it's on the right windward side. Alternatively turn the board and sail the other way.

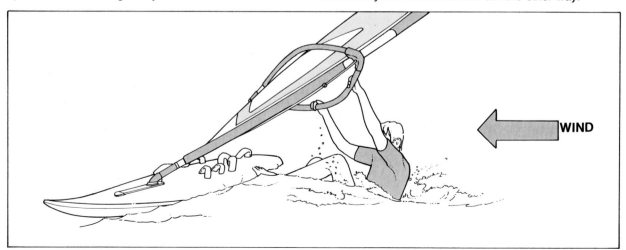

5.. On a beam to broad reach you can reach the tail and tuck your back foot into one of the back straps for a firm foothold. Then bend your back leg to bring your body close in to the board. The closer you are, the more the rig will be upright and able to catch the wind. In light airs, you need to be very close to the board.

you can get both hands on the boom in the sailing position, but until you reach this stage you must continue to swim the rig forward.

Powering the Sail

As soon as your back hand is on you can sheet in and give some power to the sail which will be enough to keep it forward, but don't overdo this or you will find the rig is torn from your grasp.

Get the feel of power in the rig while lying in the water. Sheeting in on the back hand will make the board bear way on to a beam reach course, which is what you need to complete the waterstart.

When the board is at the right angle off the wind, you should be able to reach the tail with your back foot – slip it in one of the back straps for a firm foothold. You can then bend your back leg up under your chin to bring the tail in towards you.

Getting Lift from the Wind

Straighten your arms above your head so that the rig is as upright as possible and will catch maximum lift from the wind. Wait for a suitable gust which feels strong enough to pull you all the way up. When it comes, stand up on your back leg while kicking hard with the other until you can get it up on to the deck. All the time keep sheeted in to prevent the board luffing, before sailing away.

Once you've got the hang of it, the waterstart is as easy as riding a bicycle. In light winds it can be hard, and it's important to get your body in close to the board.

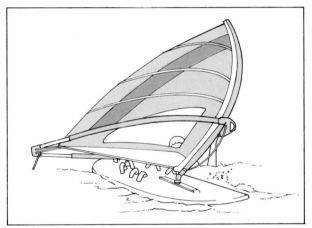

3. Get the nose of the board facing into the wind and the mast at right angles. This is the easiest position for pulling the rig up from the water by tugging on the mast.

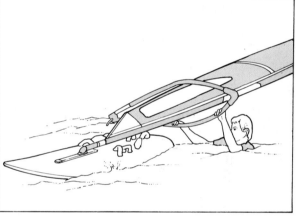

4. Get the feel of the power in the rig by sheeting in and out with your back hand. Sheeting in will make the board bear away until you can reach the tail.

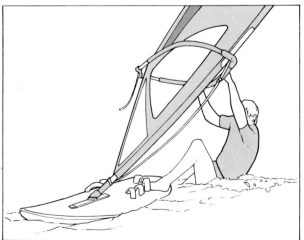

6. Wait for a suitable gust which will pull you up. When it comes tread water with your front foot, stand up on your back leg, and put your weight on the mastfoot.

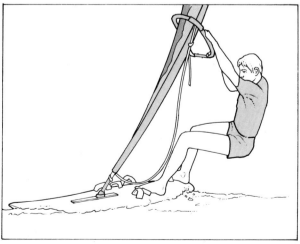

7. Stand up fully so you can get your front foot into the strap. The board may tend to luff up, so sheet in and if necessary rake it forwards to counteract this.

Gybing

On a short board, the only gybe to do is a carve gybe which is carried out at full planing speed. It is a more difficult technique than waterstarting or basic jumping and takes much effort to learn. Once mastered, though, it's a very satisfying and effective manoeuvre.

You should be good at doing a basic carve gybe on a 295 before you tackle it on a shorter board. These are prone to stall because of their lack of volume. Once you're proficient at the basic carve you can attempt variations such as one-handers, duck gybes, and scissor gybes (see pages 74–79).

The Basic Carve
Good conditions for gybing are a Force 4 wind and fairly flat water, although a well formed wave which will help you maintain speed during the gybe is useful.

The board must plane effortlessly, but not be going so fast that you lack control and the skeg is starting to slide. If it is, you must sheet out to throttle back a little.

If there's a small wave to bank off this can help the manoeuvre since you won't have to concentrate so much on keeping the board moving.

Starting the Gybe
To start the gybe, take your back foot out of the strap and position it so that your toes are just over the inner rail. Pull up on the front foot and weight the back so that the board begins to carve away from the wind rapidly.

Lean in towards the sail while sheeting in to the angle of the wind, all the time concentrating on carving a smooth and fairly gradual turn – no sudden movements to upset the board's momentum.

Changing to the New Tack
The board will continue to carve round through the eye of the wind and on to the new tack. You will know when you need to gybe because your back hand will start to pull hard – that's the time to let go, and transfer it to the mast.

Continue to carve (you need to be able to do this automatically) and with your other hand taken away from the boom the rig will flip round of its own accord.

Catch it on the new side, and then shift your front foot to flatten the board and straighten out its course before it rounds up too far into the wind.

Finally, move your feet to their positions for the new reach, move your hand from mast to boom and sail off – maintaining good speed throughout for a perfect gybe!

Right: The board should be carved in one easy motion all the way through 180 degrees. Only then do you stop carving, and move your feet into the new straps (**8**).

Getting used to having your feet the wrong way round takes time, as your body is contorted and twisted until you are ready to straighten out the board.

If you can find a wave to keep up your speed it will make the middle and final parts of the gybe much easier, so that you can concentrate on getting the rig to flip (**5–7**) through hand control and gradual carving, while the wave keeps the board moving. It requires much practice for a totally fluid movement.

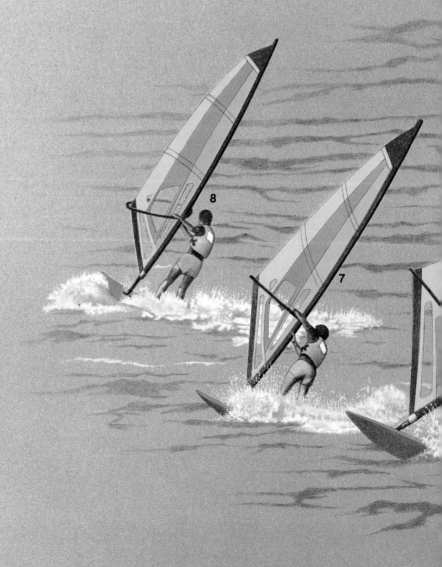

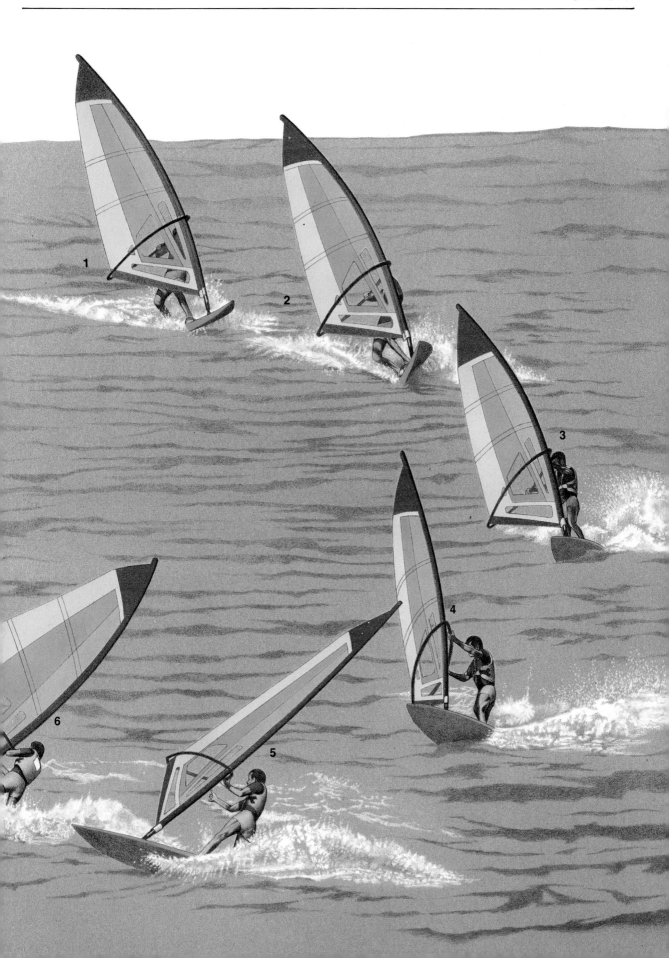

Spin-out

Spin-out occurs when air gets around the fin, and the tail suddenly slides out from under you. It usually happens at high speed, particularly if there is chop making the tail of the board bounce on and off the water.

Putting even bigger fins on is not the answer, and it will make you slow down. Get used to a style of sailing with your weight off the fin and directed on to the mastfoot. The sail should have the centre of effort well forward with minimum pull on the back end of the boom.

Tail Slide
If the tail starts to slide, dig in the leeward rail and bear off until the spin-out stops. If you are spinning-out a lot, this makes getting upwind quite difficult. The only other way to avoid this is to slow the board right down.

You can experiment with various strap, fin, and mastfoot positions for optimum trim without spin-out. If that doesn't work your board may be at fault; for instance, a very flat tail with little V or rocker will be prone to spin-out.

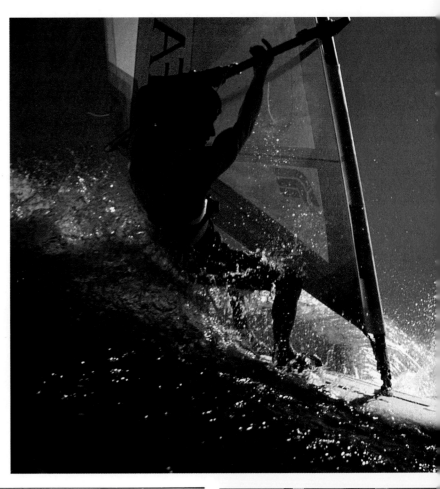

Sailing Upwind

Sailing a short board upwind is a compromise between going for speed and pointing.

A low volume board must be kept planing fast for maximum lift to windward from the skeg. This will allow you to close reach upwind fairly effectively.

Sailing Stance
The sailing stance is similar to that used on a long board, with your body leaning forward into the direction of travel and the rig sheeted into the centreline.

No short board is effective upwind, but some are better than others. The most important factor is often the tide, and if you are sailing in a tidal area you should have a clear notion if it is taking your board upwind (good) or downwind (bad). This is what makes a location such as Columbia Gorge (page 130) ideal.

Marginal Conditions
In light winds when it's difficult to sustain planing on a close reach, you will need to push the windward rail deep in the water with your weight well forward. This will extend the waterline length of the board to its maximum, so that it behaves like a long daggerboard. Obviously this technique becomes more difficult and less successful with low volume boards.

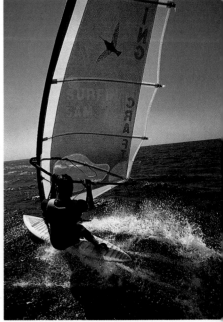

When the Wind Drops

Weight placement becomes critical in marginal planing conditions. Pumping the rig back and forward helps gain speed, but is wasted unless board trim is good. Try to keep it level from rail to rail, with your weight forward and off the tail. If the board shows any tendency to drop off the plane you must lean your weight forward on to the mastfoot.

If the wind drops right away your problems will depend on your board and your weight. Gary Gibson in the photo below has obviously underestimated his board size for the prevailing conditions, and his only solution is to swim home.

You must learn to waterstart in the lightest winds to avoid this situation. Start with your front hand on the mastfoot, and once up keep well forward.

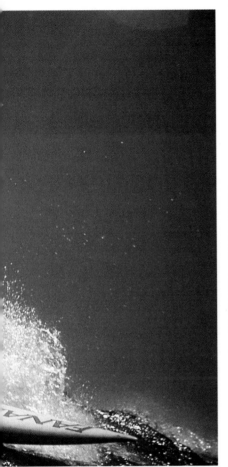

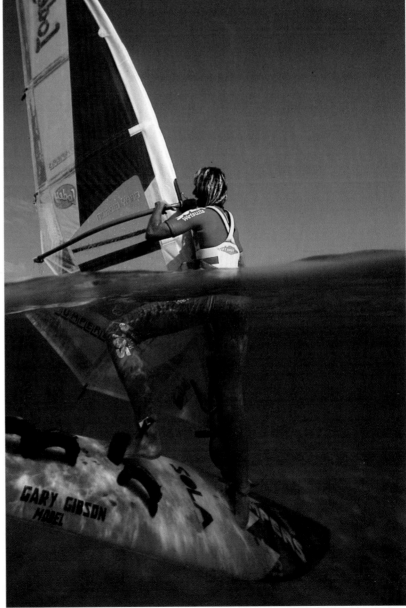

Above: Coming in with the waves at high speed there should be no spin-out problems if the tail is firmly in the water. However, going out through waves or sailing through chop will cause the tail to jump in and out of the water, and that's when spin-out is most likely to happen.

Left: Good stance for sailing upwind. The sailor twists his body and leans forward with the rig well sheeted in. Planing in a marginal wind, the windward rail is weighted for extra lateral resistance against going sideways.

Right: This is what they call a sinker! When the wind drops you have no way of sailing home on a sinker. You can't waterstart, can't uphaul, and even if you could, the board would be submerged underneath you.

Jumping Waves

When you're sailing on the open sea, there will invariably be waves unless there is no wind or it's blowing offshore – both are useless for your needs!

The fastest way to reach out is to avoid jumping, flexing your legs like a ski racer to take the board over the waves without leaving the surface of the sea.

However, any short board is only too willing to get airborne if you will let it do so. Its speed and light weight will send it skywards whenever it hits a ramp.

Using Small Waves
To start with try using small crumbly waves which will be fairly forgiving, and avoid any that have heavy, dumping, white water. Look for the steepest part, and head for it at maximum speed but under full control with two-thirds of your weight resting on your front foot.

As the nose of the board meets the wave, put your weight on to your back foot, sheet in, and un-weight the board by flexing your legs as the tail leaves the wave.

When you reach the apex of the jump kick the tail upwind of the nose so that the board is heading off downwind and will not spin-out when it lands. Do this with your legs partly flexed to absorb the shock, and land tail first with the sail sheeted in for support.

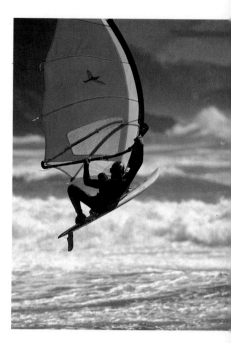

Right: Jumping puts a lot of sideways strain on the skeg which must be strong enough not to break out on landing.

Flat Water Jumps

If you've built up enough speed, it's possible to make jumps of over a metre (up to four feet) from virtually flat water.

This is great for adding some variety to reaching up and down on inland waters, and if there's any chop present (or a wake from a motorboat) it's possible for a top sailor to get a complete upside-down jump.

Making the Jump
The main requirements for a jump are power and sufficient control. You will need winds in the 20–30 knot range, and should carry a sail which is just controllable, although overpowered in gusts.

To start, the board must be at full speed and under control on a beam reach. To learn this tech-nique look for some suitable chop to launch the board from. Stand upright, both knees slightly flexed and ready. The picture sequence on the right, numbered 1 to 3, shows how to tackle the jump.

1. Just before hitting the chop, luff the board a little by weighting the inner rail. Put your weight on your back foot, and as the nose hits the chop sheet in hard and pull up with your front foot. This will expose the windward bottom side of the board for maximum lift.

2. Keep sheeted in, crouch down and then flex both legs to pull the board up under your body so that it is level and in mid air.

3. Prepare for landing by sheeting out slightly and increasing pressure on the front foot to reduce the chance of a spin-out. Flex your legs so that they act as shock absorbers. Keep your weight off the back foot so the tail doesn't slide away on impact. Sheet in, stand up, and sail away. If you're good, you can do all this with surprisingly little loss of speed.

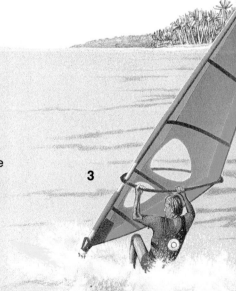

3

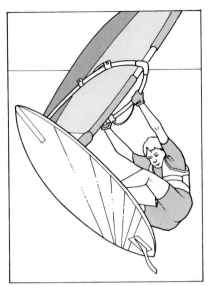

1. Sheeted in just after take off. The legs are flexed, and pushing the nose downwind for landing.

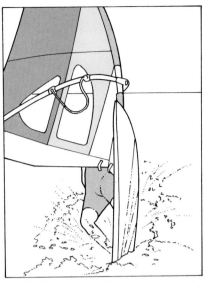

2. Swing the board under your body to land tail first which is less likely to damage your board.

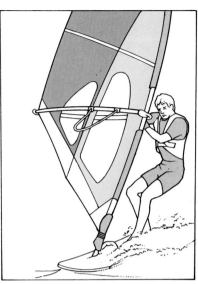

3. Beware of spin-out at this point. Shift your weight on to your front foot to get it off the tail.

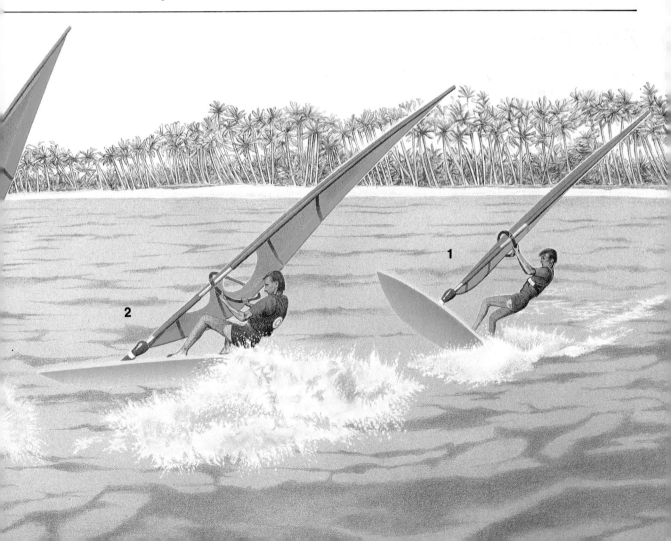

Advanced Technique

Having mastered the basics of handling a short board, this section takes you through to more advanced techniques which you can use on short boards ranging in size from a 295 to a sinker.

Now is the time you will be thinking of moving on to a second, smaller short board which will give you a better response and control in really strong winds. The popular

Below: Stuart Sawyer is halfway through an aerial gybe, using a Vitamin Sea custom board.

Vitamin Sea is one of the best known British custom brands, run by Tad Ciatula and based in England's West Country, which has a strong surfing tradition.

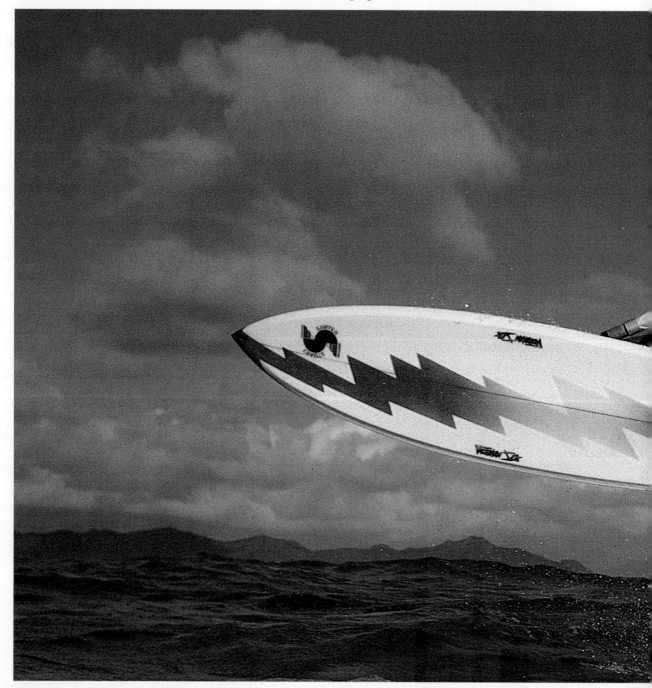

The board shown is 2.60 m (8 ft 6 in) and weighs about eight kilos (17 lbs). It is built in the classic custom materials of Clarkfoam and a polyester resin laminate, with double stringers for maximum stiffness and strength. However, all custom boards are fragile and need careful handling. length is around 2.70 m (8 ft 10 in), though you can go as short as 2.45 m (8 ft). Take care that you don't try to run before you can walk!

Choice in production boards is limited, so this is a great opportunity to 'go custom'. A custom board should give you exactly what you want and may give you a chance to work out your own design ideas.

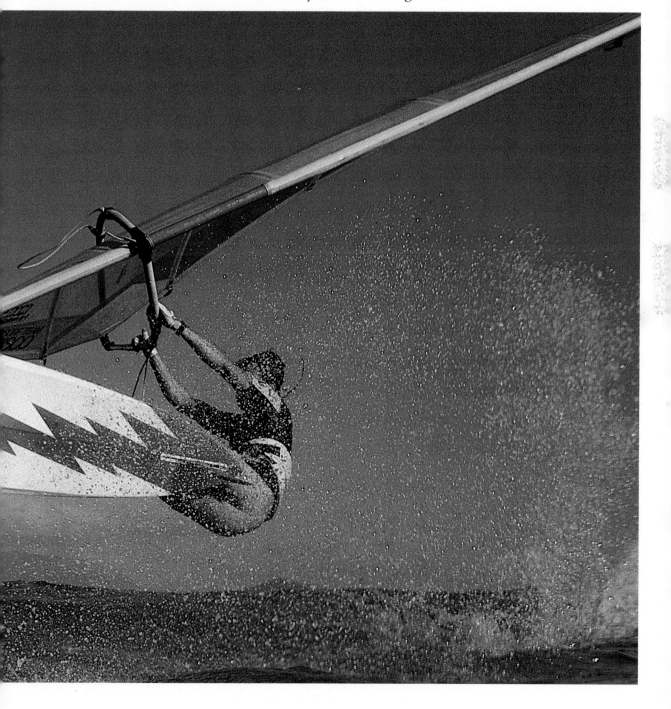

One-handed Carve Gybe

Although it has no real practical value, the one-handed carve gybe is popular among short board freestylists and does help to develop co-ordination and fluidity. Casually trailing a hand in the water while carving a perfectly controlled gybe also looks very good from the beach!

To start with you need flat water and enough wind to keep your board planing fast when carrying a 5.50 sq m (59 sq ft) sail.

1. While sailing fast on a close reaching course, check to leeward to make sure it's clear. Then take your back foot out of the strap and press down with your toes close to the inside rail, leaning into the turn with knees bent and pulling up on the front strap.

2. While controlling the radius of the turn with your foot pressure, release your back hand from the boom and reach for the water while bending your knees more and leaning more into the turn.

3. Score maximum points by leaving your hand trailing in the water until the last possible second, before reaching for the boom on the new side with what has become your new front hand. Don't attempt to put your front hand in the water too early, you will lose too much speed and may stall the board. In addition, if you leave it too late, you will probably stall and fall in to windward instead of sheeting in and powering away.

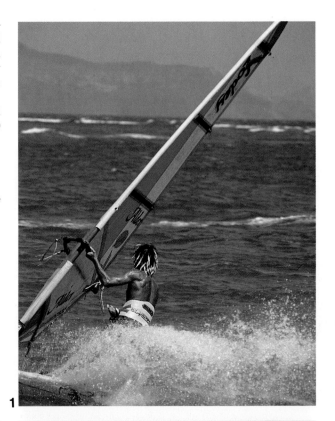

1

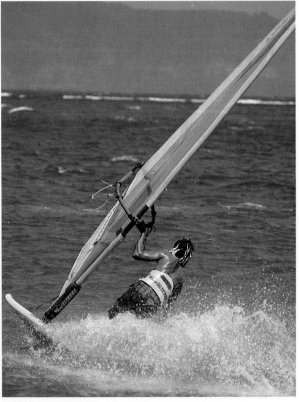

2

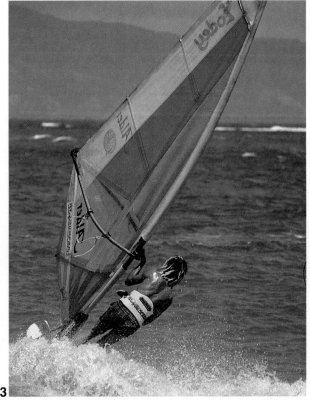

3

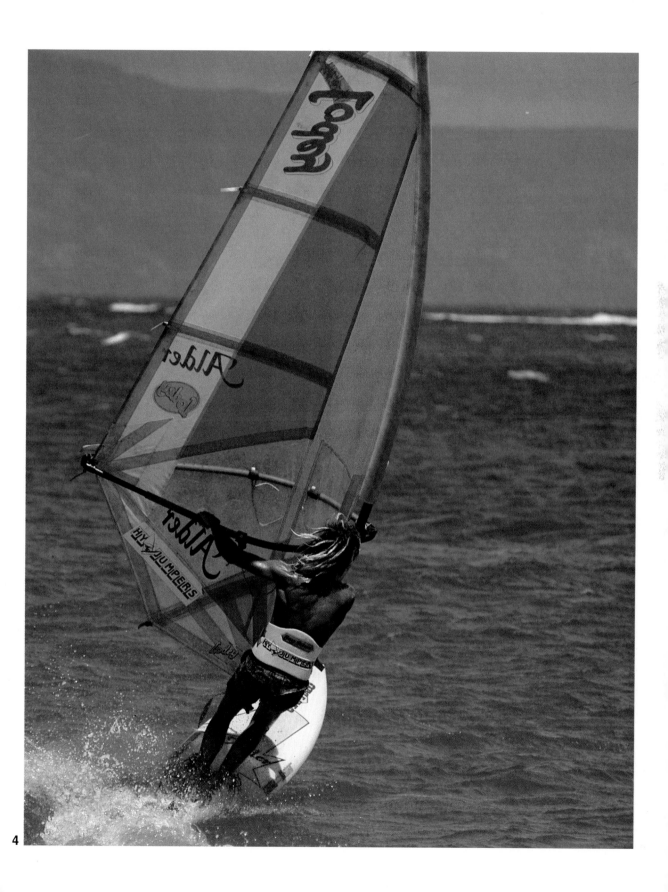

Duck Gybe

This stylish alternative to the ordinary carve gybe was developed by Hawaiian sailor Richard Whyte back in 1981. Since that time it has caught on to the extent that it is now part of almost every proficient short board sailor's repertoire of flashy manoeuvres, as shown here by Gary Gibson. Before attempting the duck gybe, your conventional carve gybes should be expert to the degree where the exits are almost as fast as the entries.

1. While sailing fast on a reach, check that no one is in the way and then take your foot out of the back strap to steer into the gybe. Control the turn by foot pressure, and take your front hand off the boom so that the rig falls downwind.

2. Immediately grab the end of the boom behind your back hand; and then let go with the back hand so that you can pull the rig over your head and reach for the new boom, all the time remembering to keep carving through the turn.

3. Having caught the new boom with the old back hand, quickly follow with the old front hand.

4. Finally, switch your feet, sheet in, and sail away on the new reach with the duck gybe successfully completed. Bear in mind that premature sheeting in before the board is completely carved round may catapult you over the nose.

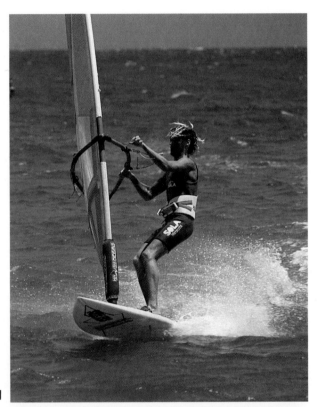

1

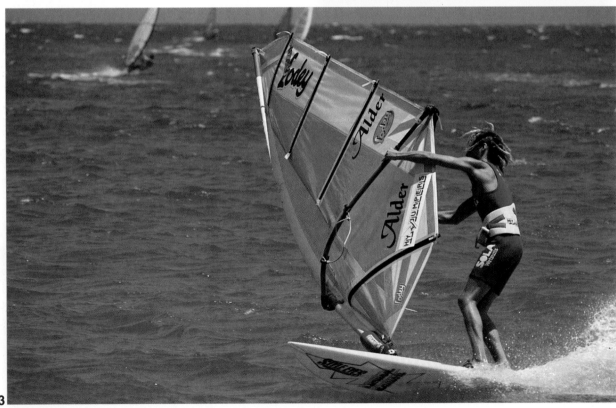

3

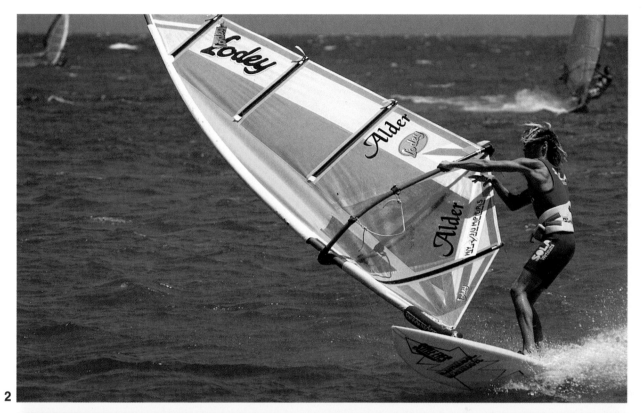

2

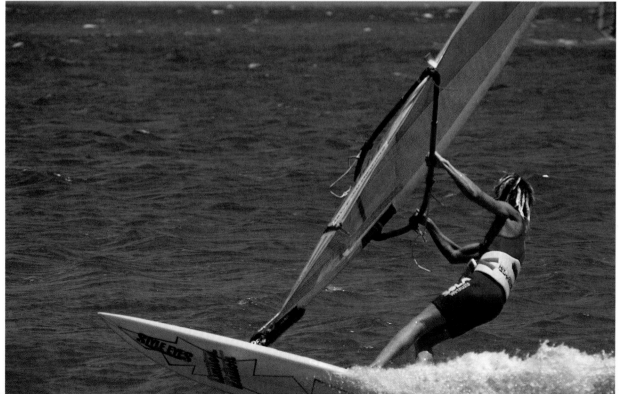

4

Scissor Gybe

This relatively new gybing style is now commonplace amongst the world's most expert wave and slalom sailors. The object is to make a rapid turn-around while losing minimum ground downwind, and unlike the regular carve gybe it does not necessitate keeping the board planing throughout the radius of the manoeuvre. This makes it particularly important in a slalom competition where you may need to crack your board round a mark inside another competitor, since you don't have to use as much room as you do to carve round in the usual style.

Scissor Gybe Technique

The scissor gybe in these photos is demonstrated by Farrell O'Shea, sailing in Hawaii.
1. Excessive speed makes the scissor gybe impossible, so just before the turn you should be planing, but not breaking speed records! As with a conventional gybe start the turn by bearing away in the usual style.
2. Suddenly lift hard with your front foot, and simultaneously push the leeward (inside) rail down and away from you with the back foot. The effect of this is to make the board kick its nose up in the air.
3. With the nose clear of the water the board spins round on its tail section. You are now totally committed and must remain so, keeping your knees bent and crouching to maintain a low centre of gravity so that you can keep your balance. In an instant the board will spin round so that you find yourself with the sail clew-first and your legs crossed – which is why it's called the 'scissors'. If you've kept your balance you can now change your feet to their new positions, let the rig flip, and sail off on the new tack.

To start with you should practise the manoeuvre in light airs when it's easier to control the rig clew-first. Once you become more competent the scissor gybe can be accomplished in higher winds, becoming increasingly more radical and difficult. This gybe is vital for successful slalom racing; and it's also worth being able to handle the scissor gybe if you want to make a snappy gybe in front of a big wave, or just want to keep yourself up to windward while out sailing.

You can control the speed of the scissor with your feet – if you scissor them across one another speedily the board will turn really fast.

A similar technique can be used on a long board, but because of its greater length and weight of the hull it relies much more on the rig, and is usually called the 'pivot' gybe, with the sailor jumping on the tail to bring the board to a dead halt, and then using the rig to pivot the board around in its own length. Alternatively the 'flare' gybe is accomplished by sinking the tail and weighting the windward outer rail, and is at its fastest with the daggerboard fully down and mastfoot right back.

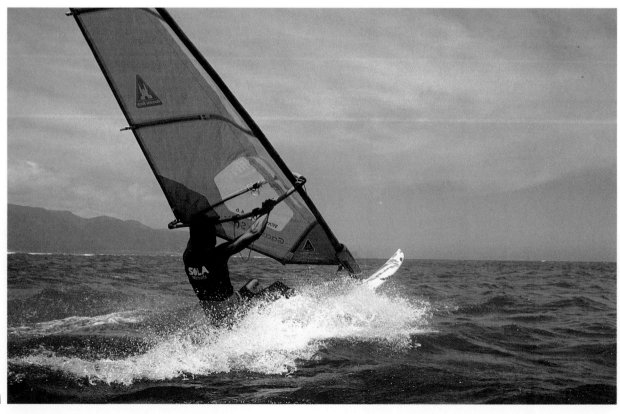

1

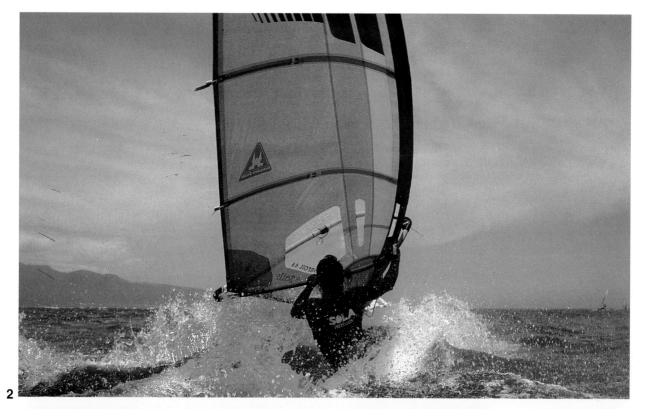

2

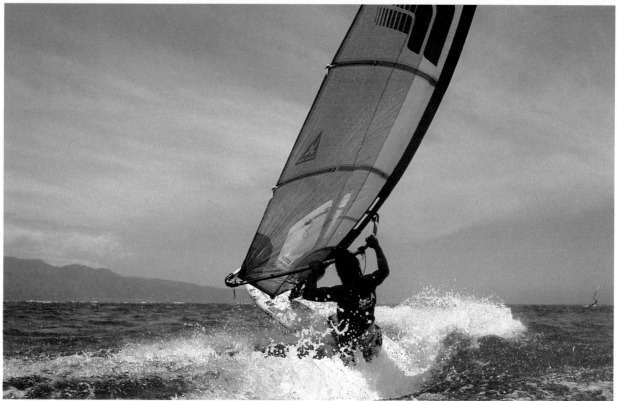

3

Aerial Gybe

The aerial gybe is one of the most radical manoeuvres in the repertoire and first appeared in 1985. It involves jumping, carve gybing, body dragging, and a very agile sailor.

It's helpful to make use of a small wave. Sail along at maximum speed, take your back foot out of the strap, and at the right moment lean the rig back, pull up hard on the front foot, and immediately take the weight off your back foot.

Taking Off

As the tail leaves the water (1), concentrate on pulling it into the wind with your toes curled round the top of the strap for extra grip. The board should be in flight and about horizontal as it starts to head more downwind.

The next stage (2) is harder. You have to get your body lower than the board; get the tail of the board higher than the nose; and start to *push* the tail round by sliding your foot forward on the board (3).

Landing

As you come in to land there are three points to remember:
1. The nose is lower than the tail, because you are pivoting the board around it.
2. Your back foot is near level with your front foot, and also on the rail.
3. The board has passed the dead downwind point.

At this stage the board is going sideways and backwards, and it's vital that you keep your foot well forward and over the new windward rail to stop both tail and rail digging in.

On landing you are in the clew-first position (4), and there's a tremendous amount of torque as the board's momentum is halted while you're being pulled forward. Nifty footwork is needed to control the sail and prevent you being launched (5).

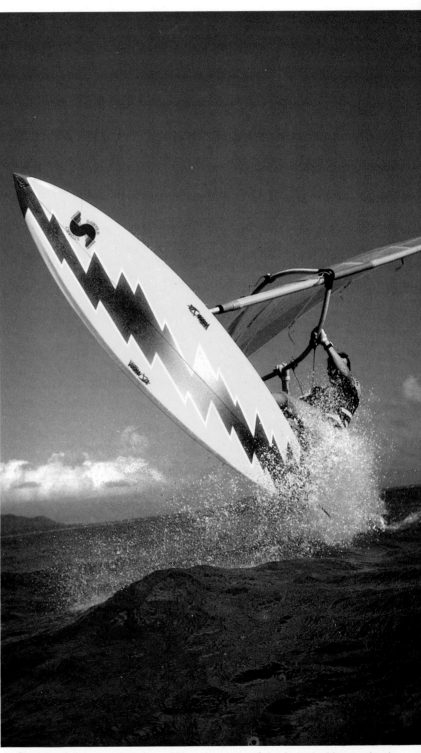

1. Start as if doing a chop hop, lifting the nose of the board with your back foot out of the strap. Concentrate on making the tail of the board weightless so that it jumps well clear, while trying to lift it up and into the wind (blowing from right to left in all pictures).

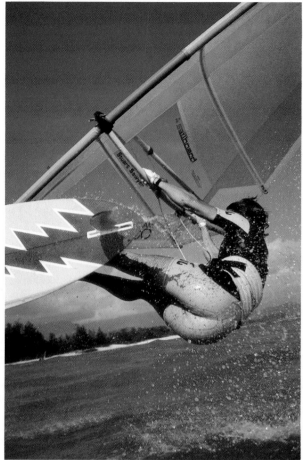

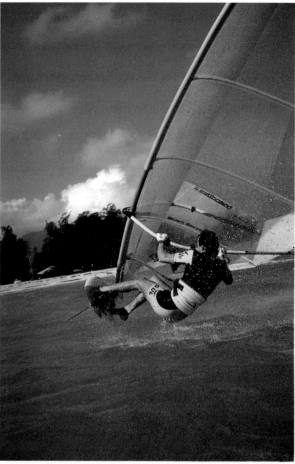

2. Hold your toes over the back strap, and try to get the board higher than your body, with its tail higher than the nose. Push the board around until it's pointing further and further downwind.

3. At this point you are almost cross-legged. Slide your back foot forward and well over the rail which will allow you to push the tail upwards as well as around, ready for a good landing.

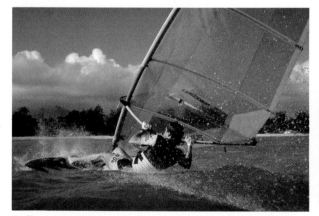

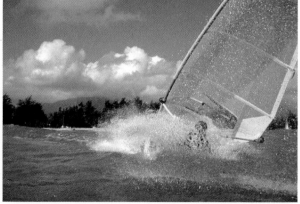

4. Try and get the nose to land first, so as to pivot the board around it. To combat the torque from board and rig, it helps to let your body drag a little while pressuring the windward rail.

5. Allow the sail to pull you upright with the old front foot acting as an anchor. You can then flip the rig, change foot positions, and sheet in for the new tack. Performed by Stuart Sawyer.

Body Drag

Do you sail your short board in a warm climate where you have problems keeping cool? If so, the body drag is a trick which is worth learning. It not only cools you down, but it looks very good, as Stuart Sawyer shows here.

The main requirement is enough wind to get your board planing really fast. Force 5 is about right, and your sail should be a little oversize for easy handling. If it's not big enough, it won't have the necessary power required to drag you through the water.

Walking on Water
Go as fast as possible, and step out of the straps while blasting along. To begin the drag, step on the water lightly with your front foot. This will be dragged back towards the tail of the board immediately. Keep your toes stretched out straight so that your foot just skips along the surface.

Bend your back leg, and put your weight on to the rig and on to the water through your front hand and leg. When your weight has been taken (this all happens at once), you can step off with your back foot. Now both legs are dragging, keep your toes pointed and

the tops of your feet should aquaplane.

Keep your back hand sheeted in to maintain speed and control from the sail – you could be launched by the rig at this stage and there are no footstraps to save you.

The duration of the drag will depend on the wind and board speed, but a safe time is from two to five seconds. As soon as you start to sink it's time to get back on. If you leave it until your body stops planing you will simply drag the board to a halt.

Back on Board
To get back on the board, twist your body so that most of your weight on the water is concentrated on your front leg. Pull up with your back hand and lift your back leg up on to the board in one move. When your foot is firmly on the deck use the boom to pull you up into a standing position, lifting your front leg up and on to the deck. At the same time continue to blast along in a straight line on your reach.

Below: Ultimate cool off! Here the body drag is demonstrated to perfection by Stuart Sawyer.

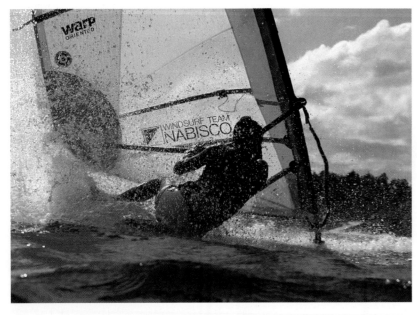

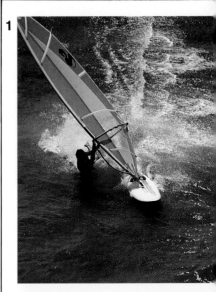
1

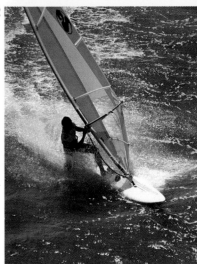
2

1. Don't leave getting back on the board too long, or your body will cease to plane and start to act with the efficiency of a bucket being dragged along through the water!

2. Careful control of the rig is vital to prevent yourself being launched and to keep on a straight course, before pulling down on the boom with your back hand and stepping back on to the board with your back foot.

3. Back on course for straight line blasting between body drags.

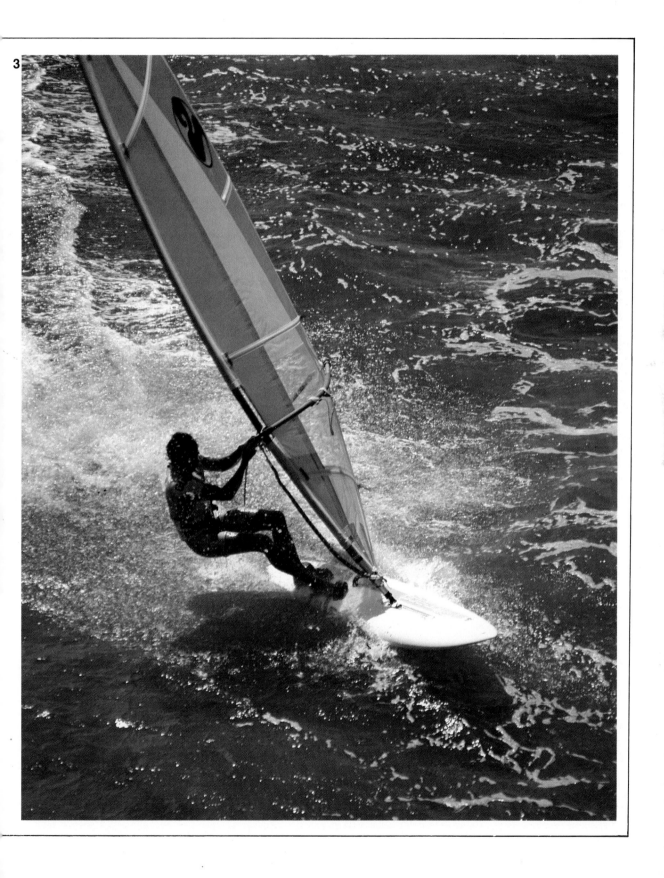

Clew-first Waterstart

The most frequent falls occur when gybing, and then lots of time is wasted trying to get going again. This often spoils what could have been a great beam reach, turning it into a hard work close reach, as you pinch up to get the board back to your start point.

If you take a tumble in mid-gybe, however, you may be able to keep holding on to the boom. You can then waterstart clew-first, and flip the rig round the right way once you're up on the board and moving. This is really the quickest and smartest looking way of getting going again.

Practice Falls
In strong winds or gusts the clew-first waterstart can be well nigh impossible. It is always tricky anyway unless you have a rig with a very short boom.

The best way to learn is to fall off deliberately and give yourself plenty of practice. Go for a gybe, bearing off through the eye of the wind, and at that point catch the rail and fall in on what is the new windward side.

Get your feet off the board so that it floats level, while sheeting out the clew end of the sail with your front hand.

Put your back foot up on the board again with your front foot treading water, while you raise the rig above your head and control it

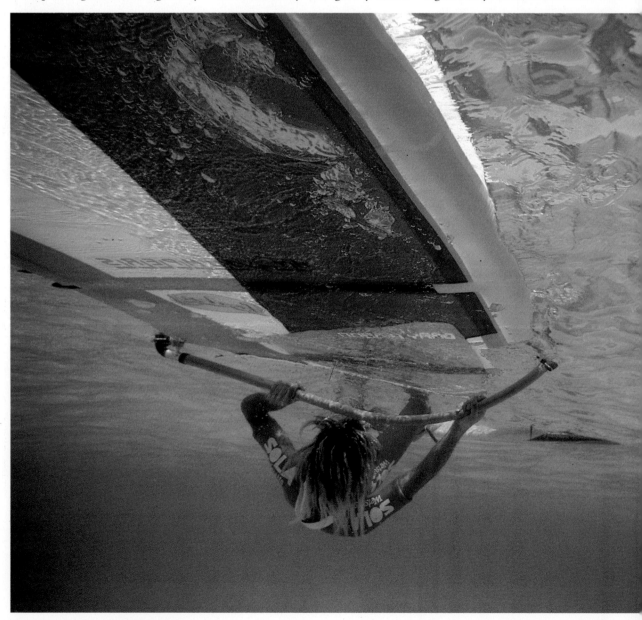

with your back (sheet) hand.

Bend your back leg to get in close to the board, and with the power in the rig stand up as with a normal waterstart. As soon as your front foot is up, let the rig flip round on to the new tack so you can sail away.

Below: Glug, glug. Few rigs will float and if you pull down you'll end up with an underwater waterstart and the luff tube full of water.

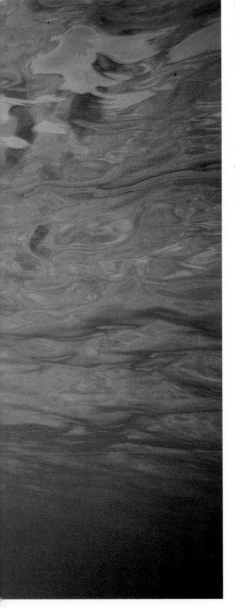

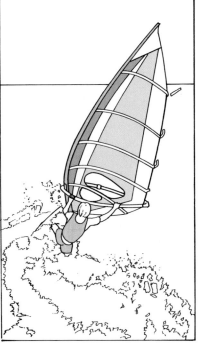

1. You've carved the board round on to the new course, but at that point it stalls and you fall in to windward, still keeping hold of the boom.

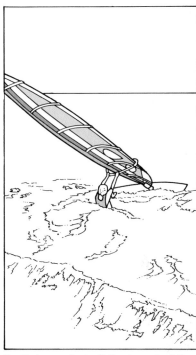

2. Get your feet off the board while sheeting out with your front hand to keep control of the rig. Then replace your back foot on the board.

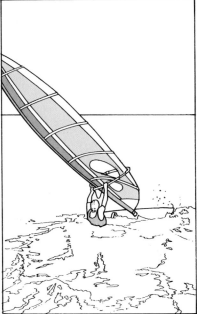

3. Raise both arms to get wind in the rig. If you lose control, let the rig flip – then you'll catch the boom the right way round to waterstart.

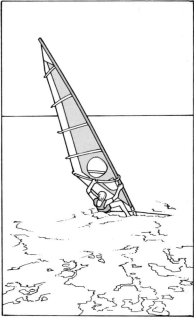

4. Bend your back leg to pull you in close to the board, and as soon as there's enough pull stand up on the board and let the rig flip round.

Helicopter Tack

Short board freestyle is a good way to improve overall fluidity when you have mastered all the variations on the carve gybe. You can practise short board freestyle in moderate winds on flat water, and then adapt it for use in a wavesailing routine. There are many variations which are possible, and the helicopter shown on these pages and the tail first tack shown overleaf are just two of the more handy tricks to be going on with.

Helicopter Technique
Apart from being very flashy and posey, the helicopter tack is also quite practical since it's a handy manoeuvre for getting upwind which allows you to change tacks without losing ground. The tail first tack is also an eye catcher, as well as being totally impractical for everyday use and extremely good for impressing the judges in a wavesailing competition.

1. Sail along on a reach, then rake the rig back and step out of the straps, bringing the board up into the head to wind position.
2. Step forward, so your front leg is just in front of the mastfoot, and really sheet in hard. This will stall the board and take you past the head to wind point.
3. At this point the sail can easily push you over into the water. Once you are past the head to wind position and oversheeted, you must be sure to resist any tendency to lean back. You can then lean forward and over the rig, pushing it over and away from you so that it fills on the leeward (bottom) side. As you do this move your front foot back behind the mastfoot.
4. Having pulled the nose of the board round through the eye of the wind by pulling the rig back, you now make it bear away on to the new tack by pushing the rig down over the front. Make sure you are standing slightly on the windward rail (left side in the photo) so that the leeward (right) rail doesn't catch and trip you.
5. As the nose turns all the way round, push the clew hard into the wind. As you do so step forward on the board so you are facing the right way. If your balance is OK you can now let the rig flip round on to the new side. If your balance is not right you can just stop and check yourself, using the rig for support.
6. When you're ready put your weight over the mastfoot and let the rig flip from clew-first to normal position. Sheet in and sail off on your new course.

Once you're proficient this manoeuvre can be done very fast on a small sinker. However, when you are learning a floaty board such as a 295 will obviously make life easier, since it won't start to wallow and sink halfway through the manoeuvre.

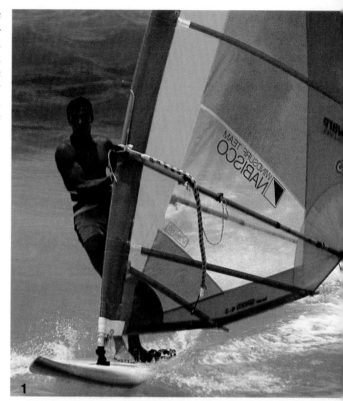

1

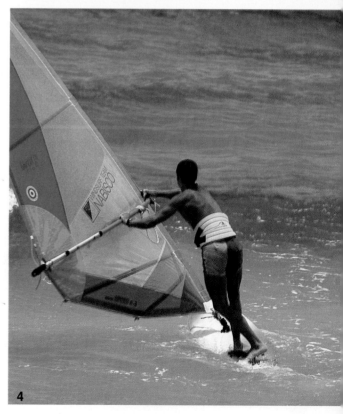

4

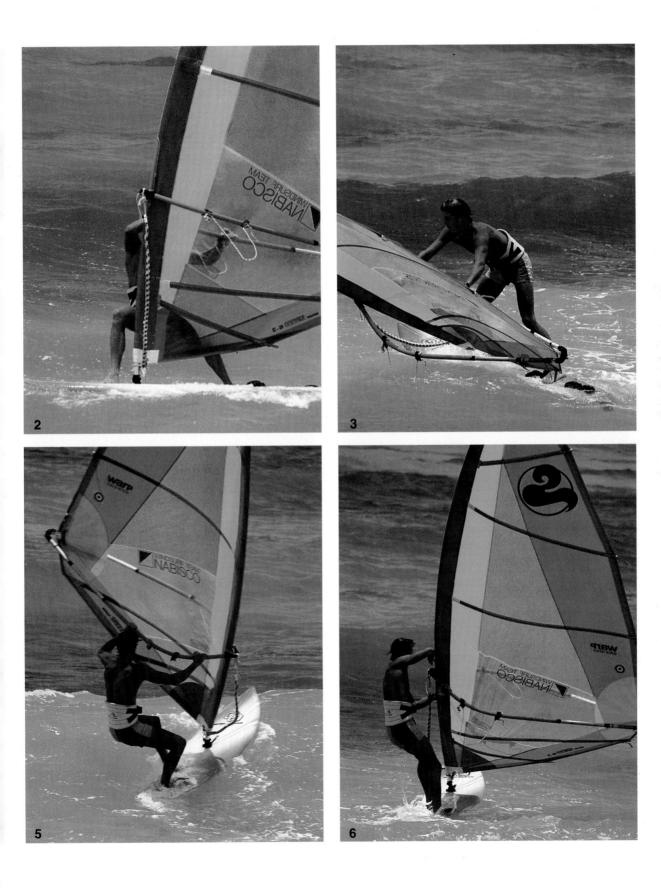

Tail-first Tack

This is an altogether more complicated transitional manoeuvre which has no particular practical use for windsurfers. But it does look exceptionally good on the water as demonstrated by Stuart Sawyer in this sequence of photos.

Tail-first Tack Technique

1. Bring the board up into the wind, sheeting in hard as you would in a helicopter tack.

2. Sheet in drastically hard to stall the board.

3. Move your front foot forward, but instead of pushing down on the rig as with the helicopter, sheet in more so that the board actually comes to a complete halt. It will then start to move backwards, and at this point you start to ease yourself on to the nose. Do this very carefully as there is no fin beneath you to prevent slip if you put too much weight on to the nose area.

4. Standing on the nose, sheet in by pulling the rig back towards you. At the same time try to lift the fin clear of the water so that the tail can pivot round on the nose until the board is on course for the new tack. With the fin clear the board will accelerate backwards, so don't lean yourself too far back at this point.
   The sail will push the board round, and as it does so you should move back on to the main part of the board. As soon as you let the fin touch the water the board will stop turning.

5. As the fin touches the water step to the middle of the board, and you will feel the tail bury as a result of the backwards momentum. At the same moment let go with your back hand so that the clew-first sail can flip round on to the new side.

6. Catch the boom on the new side and then sheet in and go. Having got through all the difficult stages, it's easy to fall in backwards during this last moment of the tail-first tack which would spoil the whole manoeuvre. With the board more or less sunk, there will be a lot of pull in the rig before it gets going.

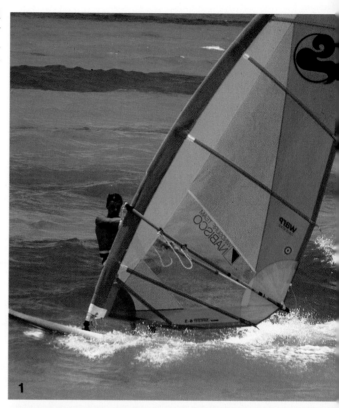

1

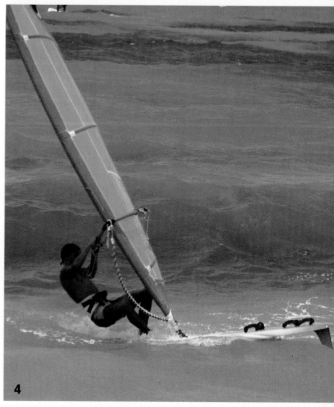

4

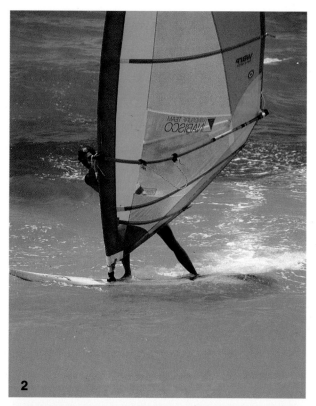

2

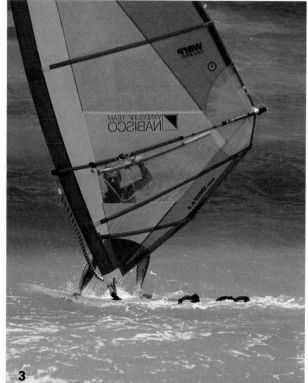

3

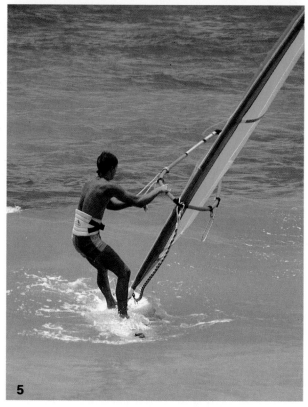

5

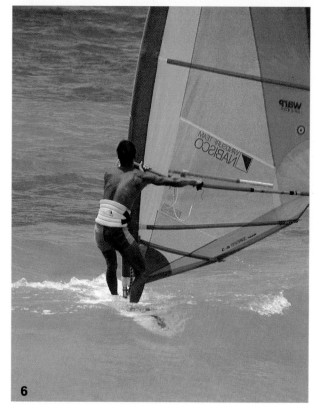

6

Wave Jumping

There are sadly few locations where there are the big ocean swells which provide the opportunities for the fully fledged kind of waveriding which is described from page 100 to 111.

However, a high performance short board can easily become airborne on the smallest of chop and when there are waves a couple of feet high they can provide enough lift for the sailor to try out the whole range of radical jumps including the loops, barrel rolls and donkey kicks which are described on the following pages.

Stresses and Strains

There is one simple rule with regard to making jumps – that is that the bigger the wave and the faster you hit it, the higher you can go.

Take note, however, that big jumps put a lot of pressure on short board equipment; in particular the mastfoot and skeg box are under enormous strain both on take-off and landing. At the point where the tail of the board is just leaving the lip there is tremendous torque on the fin if you veer to one side or the other. Also, snapping the board off the wave face before the tail has really cleared is a potential way to break off the fin.

Likewise great care must be taken on landing. The easiest way is to land so that the tail touches down first and the rest of the board follows. This spreads the impact as much as possible and absorbs the shock. More experienced sailors prefer to land nose first, which allows the board to plane out of the jump without losing too much speed. As the nose hits the water you must pull your weight back to swallow dive out of the jump – rather than just ploughing on and catapulting head first!

When Things Go Wrong

If things seem to be going sadly astray with a jump, the only answer is to bale out. When you reach the point of no return you will want to get away from your board and rig as quickly as possible, allowing them to be blown downwind where they can't land on you or you on them. Get out of the straps, push the boom away, and let go – as you go down try to remember to curl up into a ball which will make the landing as easy as possible for your poor body.

Right: Farrell O'Shea shows how to turn upside down off Hookipa, one of the few locations where conditions are good enough for both wave jumping and riding of the most exciting kind.

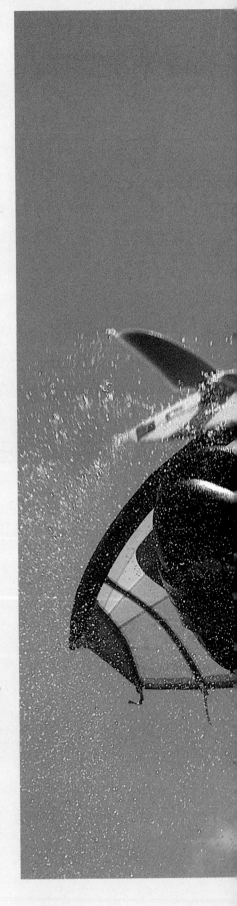

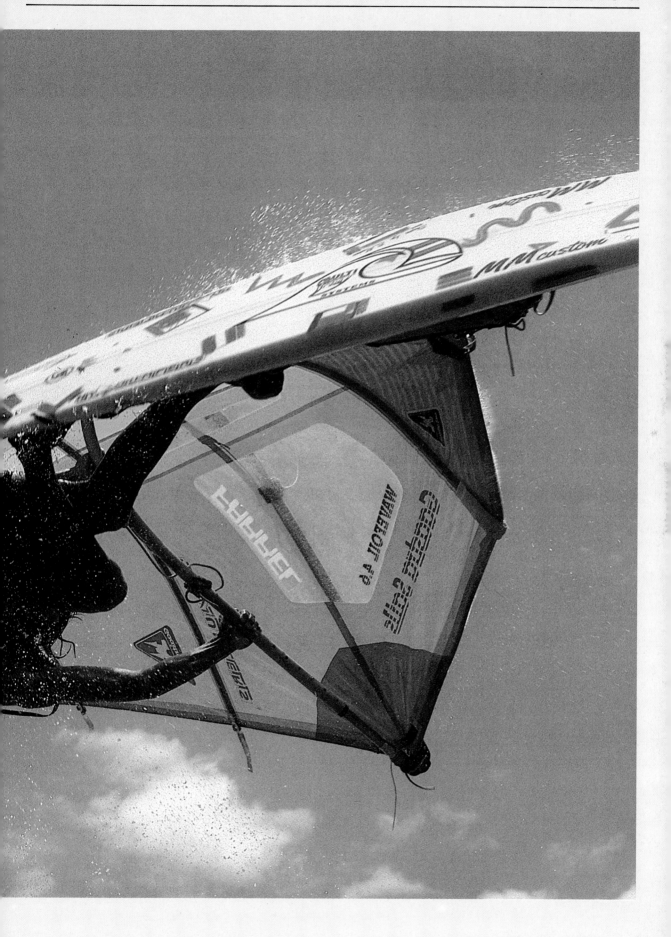

Controlled Flight

Wave Jumping

There's a big difference between hopping off waves (see pages 70–71) and the type of 'controlled flight' that can be achieved by experts – heights of over 10.5 metres (35 ft) and distances of over 15 metres (50 ft) have been recorded.

Ideal Conditions

The wind must be sideshore (or side-onshore/offshore) and sufficiently strong, but not so windy that you're having problems with control. Mushy, closely spaced waves won't give you sufficient time to get up enough speed.

You need a run-up over flat water, so that when you hit the wave your speed of 20 knots combines with its 10 knots (heading straight at you) to give a take-off speed of 30 knots!

This speed, coupled with the drop-off at the back of the wave, the steepness of the face, and successful powering of the rig, are the essentials for radical jumps.

It's surprisingly easy to break a board in half when landing. Few production boards have stringers and are therefore most susceptible to damage. Custom boards, however, can be built specifically to take this kind of hard use.

Landing

The higher or longer you jump, the harder you land, and this puts extreme sideways stress on the skeg. A large size skeg will help to counteract spin-out, but both it and the box must be strong enough not to break out on landing.

The rig must be similarly heavy-duty, and suited to the conditions. Choose a sail which is the right size and stable enough for easy control.

The Upside-downer

Maestro Robby Naish demonstrates an upside-downer off Diamond Head in Hawaii.

1. Take-off for an upside-downer must be on the steep part of the wave, the critical breaking section.

As the board leaves the lip and gains altitude, Robby kicks his back leg into the wind (blowing from left to right) while using his front foot as the board's pivot.

2. and 3. At the apex of the jump, the board is upside down and pointing into the wind with power in the rig.

4. and 5. Robby sheets in, and swings the board back under him, pressuring the back foot for a tail first landing.

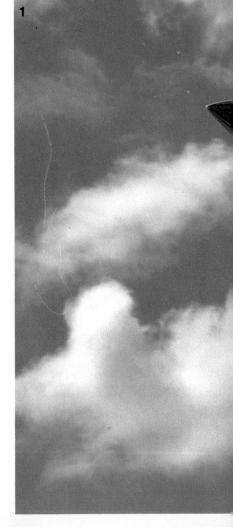

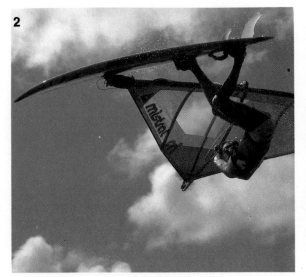

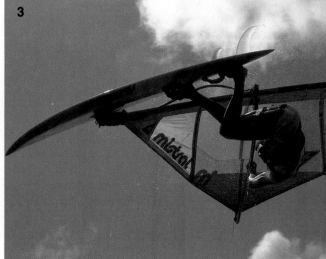

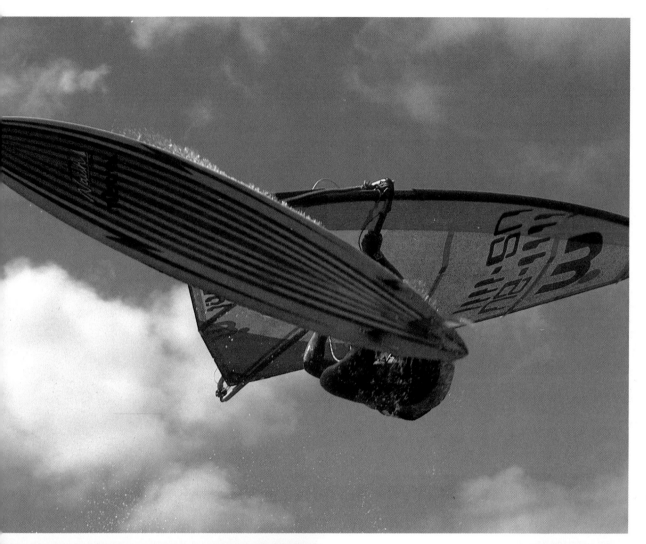

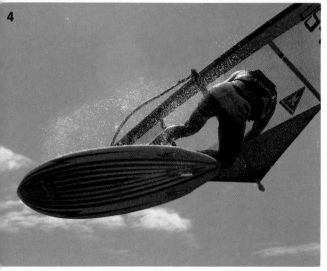

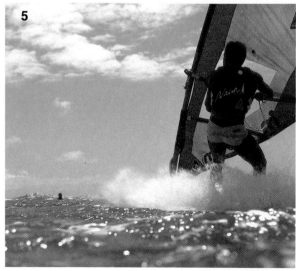

Donkey Kick

A donkey kick is an adventurous jump which actually gets you manoeuvring the board while you're up in the air. It needs a little more height from a slightly steeper wave than a basic jump, and is the start-off point for getting into really radical jumping.

It's called a donkey or mule kick, because the board is kicked out at right angles so that it's side-on to the water before coming back down to the surface and landing on its bottom.

Donkey Kick Technique

1. Approach the wave, carefully picking your spot. It's best to take off right next to the breaking part of the wave, where it is at its steepest, for a near vertical take off. Unhook as you near the wave, and crouch a little, bunching yourself up as if you're a jack-in-the-box. As the nose lifts up the wave, really jump up as you would when trying to do a straight-up jump on land. As you do so, concentrate on pulling the tail up with you.

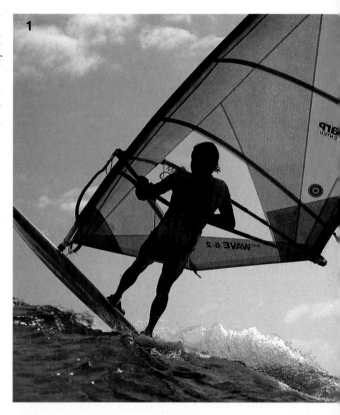

2. Twist your body towards the sail, pushing down on your back hand. This will lever your weight away from the board. As the board comes round, extend your front leg and try to push the nose out in front and slightly down. This allows you to pull your back foot under you and to the side. Your front leg will be lying almost parallel to the board.

3. The classic donkey kick position with the board kicked out side-on to the water. As you start to lose height, transfer your weight to your front hand to pull your legs back down under you. You will feel as though you are pointing downwind, but while pulling your legs down it is easy to push the tail too far, inadvertently, so that the nose comes right round into the wind. Counteracting this tendency will help to prevent spin-out on landing.

The board will tend to come down and land pretty flat, so get your legs flexed and ready to take the impact. Dropping yourself partly into the water as the board hits the surface will ease the strain on your body.

The donkey kick sequence is by Stuart Sawyer, off Red Rock beach in Barbados, using a 2.70 m (8 ft 10 in) single fin custom board.

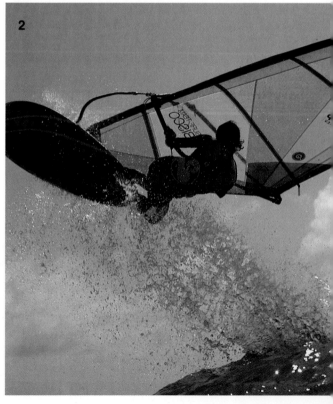

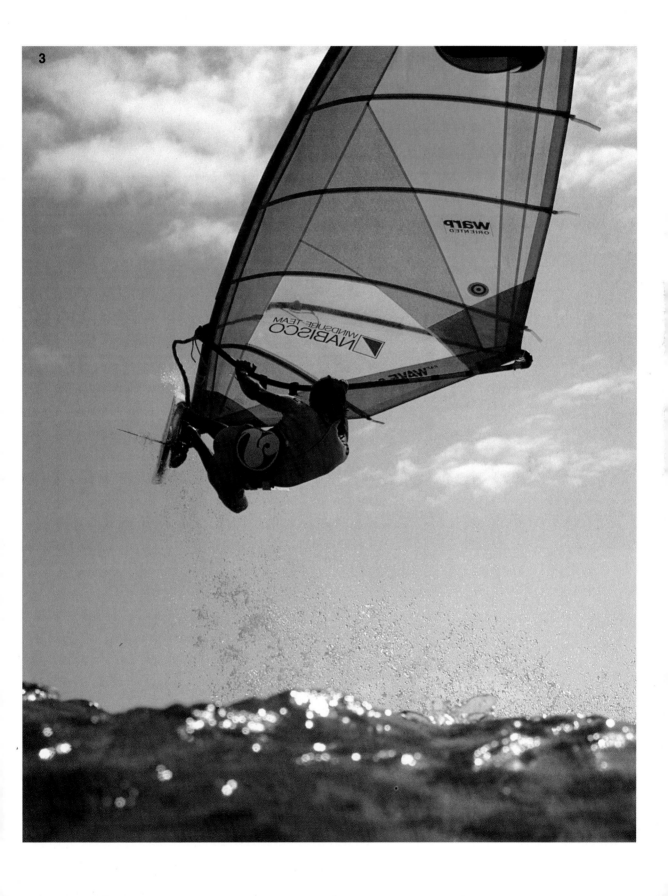

Looping

Looping your board through a 360 degree jump is certainly one of the most spectacular manoeuvres in the advanced short board sailor's repertoire! Surprisingly, it's a jump that can be performed on relatively small waves. Ideal waves are waist high with steady winds.

Basically it's an extension of an upside–down jump, which needs great speed and power in order to clear the wave with the mast tip and to continue revolving as well. This manoeuvre can, however, be extremely dangerous.

The Barrel Roll

The barrel roll is a variation which flattens the loop into a horizontal plane with the rig parallel to the water, so that not quite so much height is required to clear the mast tip and board.

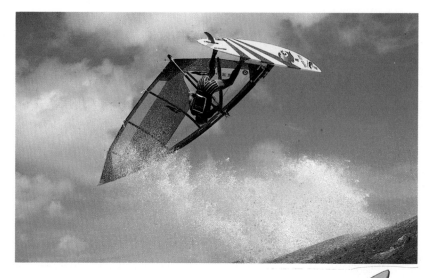

Above: Mid loop with the sailor hanging beneath his board. If things go wrong either stick with the rig and board or bale out well clear.

Looping Through 360 Degrees

1. Meet the wave at planing speed, keeping well in control. A steep ramp is essential, and you must carve the board hard round into the wind on the wave face. This will give the necessary momentum for the turn.

2. Keep the rig sheeted in throughout the loop to avoid being backwinded, while keeping it trimmed to maintain power in the sail. This is the apex of the loop – to take it beyond an upside-down jump means total commitment.

3. Coming down. Decrease pressure on the front foot and weight the tail, while still keeping sheeted in to guard against backflop.

4. Continue to weight the tail, and sheet out to the wind direction while bringing your front hand in to the body.

5. Equalize pressure on your feet and sheet out completely. The rig is now pulled over to windward to straighten the board for landing.

6. Finally, make a tail first touchdown as for an ordinary jump.

What May Go Wrong?

* If the sail backwinds after take-off it is because the rig is not sheeted in enough and the angle of attack to the wind is wrong.
* If the rig falls off to leeward before landing, you must sheet out completely and rake the rig well over to windward.
* If the board nosedives, sheet out and put more weight on the tail.
* If the mast top catches the wave, your take-off should have been more horizontal. The bigger the wave, the more vertical your take-off should be.
* Remember that wipe-outs can be painful and dangerous, damaging to both you and your board.

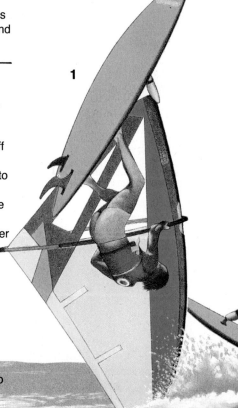

1

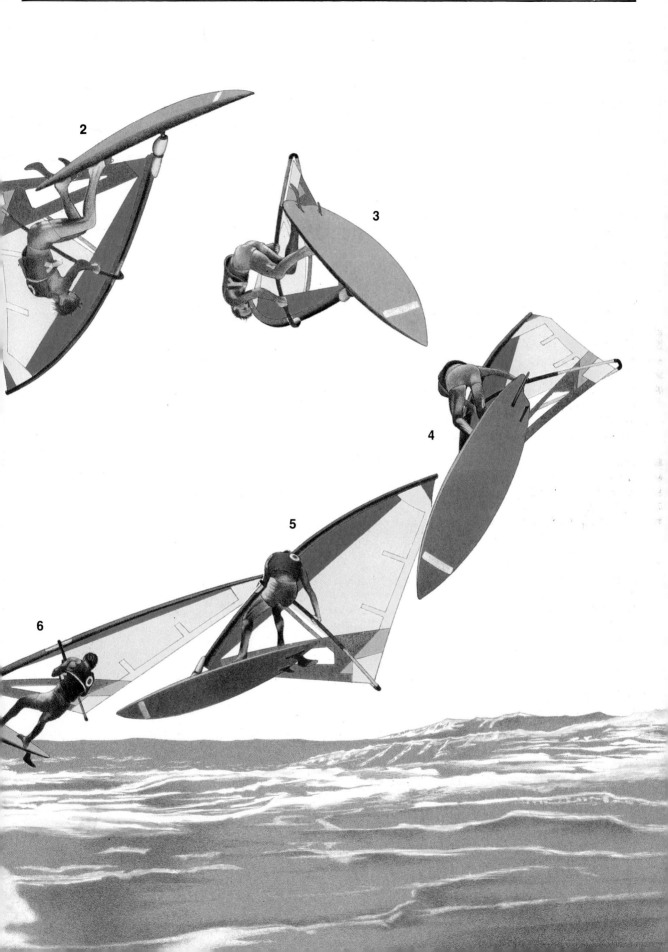

Barrel Roll

The barrel roll is a variation which flattens the loop so that not so much height is required to complete this spectacular manoeuvre.

Barrel Roll Technique

1. Pick a clean wave that's almost breaking. A clean take-off at maximum speed is essential.

2. Pull the rig back as if going into a vertical jump, but angle the nose of the board slightly into the wind. The board will reach the highest point of the roll with the sailor completely upside down, and the nose of the board and rig pointing directly into the wind before starting to come down.

3. As the board drops, push the back hand away from you to allow the clew to pass through the eye of the wind. Push the board out with your legs as the sail begins to fill — it will be very difficult to control.

4. Most attempts wipe out here! You must be confident of making nose-first landings before trying the roll.

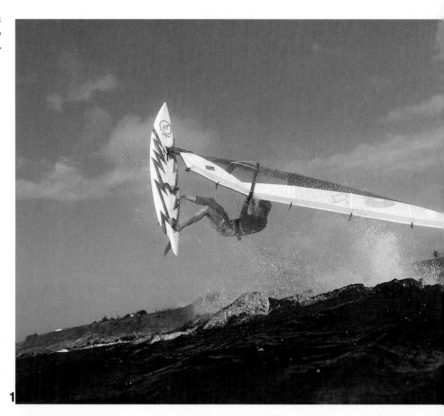

1

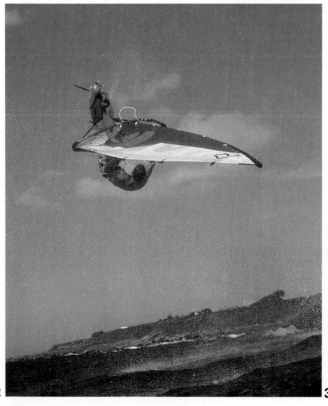

2

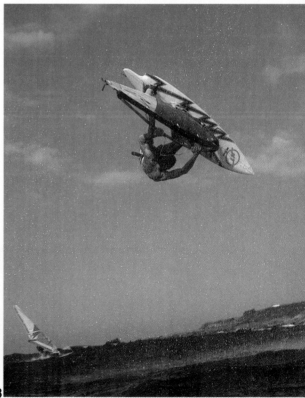

3

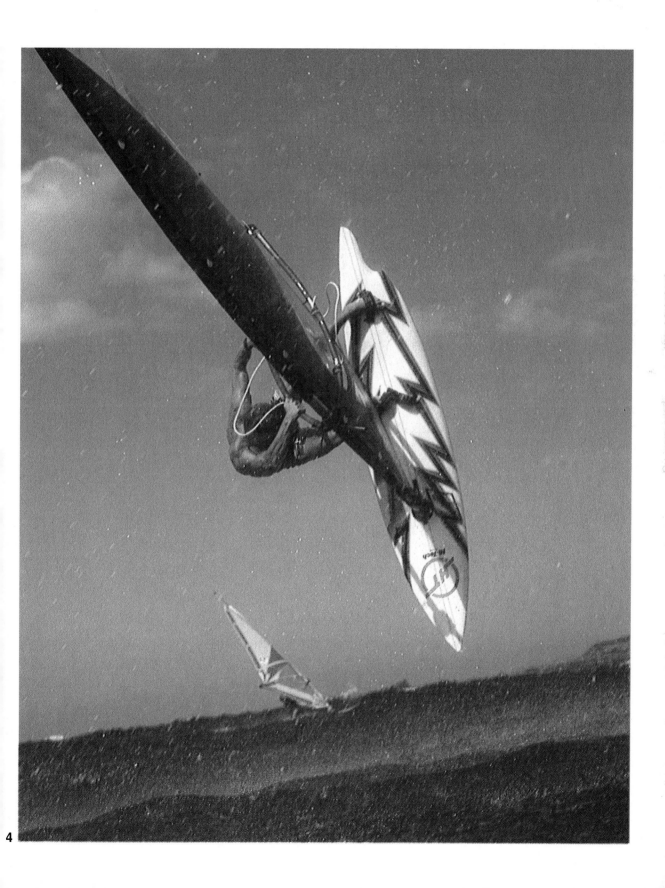

4

Big Wave Technique

The bigger the wave, the more an expert short board sailor can play on it, so long as the conditions are right for sailing. Unfortunately, most locations don't have the right kind of waves for this ultimate form of windsurfing. These perfect conditions are found in only a few corners of the world.

The Hawaiian Islands

Number One location is, of course, Hawaii, the land of surfing where the short board first developed. Hawaii benefits from waves which travel uninterrupted across the Pacific Ocean, and from Trade Winds which blow excellent Force 4 plus breezes for long periods. The summer is generally the very best season.

Diamond Head on the main island of Oahu is the best known location, immortalized by Robby Naish and the many other stars who sail there regularly. On nearby Maui the most famous spot is Hookipa which plays host to the stars and also major windsurfing events. Throughout the Hawaiian islands there are scores of similar 'ultimate' wave locations.

Other World Top Spots

Elsewhere is the world both South Africa and Australia are highly rated for potential big wave sailing. In Europe the best conditions are found along Portugal's Atlantic facing coastline, and in and around the Canary Islands which are situated just off the North African coast. All of these locations are summarized in detail in the Top Places section starting on page 124.

These select top places are wonderful for the fortunates who live there, but frustrating for those who don't and are limited to visiting them on vacation.

Luckily, however, big waves can be found in many other places but they occur on a more 'now and then' basis, depending on local wave patterns and usually demand considerable skill from the sailor. Read on to find out how to track down the big waves, and what to do when you've found them!

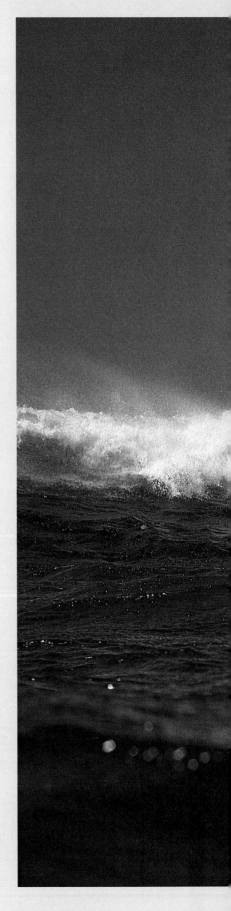

Right: Riding a wall of water is what big wave technique is all about. This is the unrivalled Robby Naish blasting his way along a wave face off the beach at Hookipa, Hawaii. Few locations offer such good waves and wind.

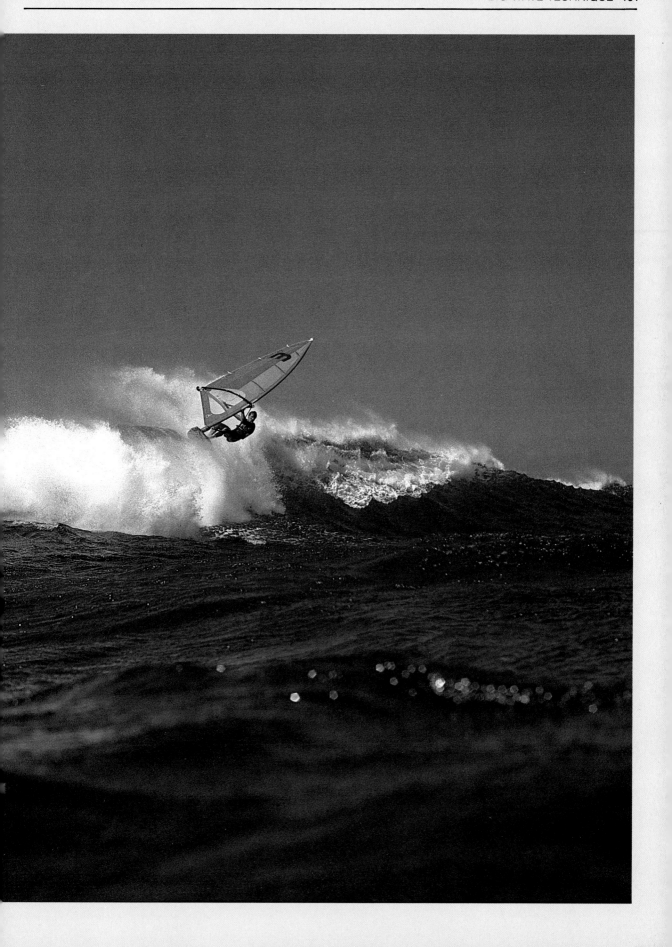

Waveriding

Choosing a Wave

On a wave face all the steering is done with feet and body movements, with speed provided as much by the steepness of the wave face as the wind in the rig.

You can ride waves anywhere that they occur, so long as they're big enough – above five foot (1.5 m) on the face (classified as 'three foot Hawaiian' as they measure them from the back) – and so long as there's sufficient wind. Force 5 is ideal, but a good sailor uses the power of the waves to sail in winds that dip below Force 4.

With a sideshore wind, you can choose your wave, waiting for the biggest one in the set before riding along its length. Wait until you catch it with the tail of your board, and then shift your weight forward (pump the rig if necessary) to help the board accelerate down the wave face.

Bottom Turns and Cut Backs

Once you hit the trough and start to lose the wave, do a 'bottom turn' to take you back up the wave face. Push down on the inner rail and handle the board and rig as you would for a carve gybe, with the momentum of your speed taking you diagonally up the face with the wind behind you. Once at the wave top (the lip) it's time for a 'cut back' to take you back down, weighting the inner rail for a sharp 90 degree turn and accelerating.

Roller Coasters

A sequence of bottom turns and cut backs can give a high speed zig-zag ride along a wave, until you lose it or it dissipates on the shore. Then you must head back out to sea to find a new wave (wave performance competition consists of 'riding' coming in, and 'jumping' going out). Either gybe on the flat water in front of the wave; or bottom turn to head up and over the wave.

1. Having accelerated down the wave, the sailor bottom turns, sheeting out and heading back up the wave face. A short boom is needed to avoid digging the end in the water.

2. He heads up the wave towards the lip, but avoids the 'critical' section where there's breaking white water as the wave crumbles.

3. To keep riding the wave, he cuts back as the board hits the lip, weighting the tail on the inner rail, and hanging out from the rig.

4. The board changes direction (a minimum 90 degrees) to head back down the wave. Sheeted in and banked hard over, the board uses the steepness of the wave face and the beam wind to hit maximum speed quickly.

5. Travelling flat out and heading for the trough of the wave. As soon as he gets in front of the wave, the sailor will go for another bottom turn, with all his weight thrown on to the inner rail. This will take him back up the wave (1), continuing until the wave breaks up and dissipates in shallow water. Two or three bottom turns and cut backs are usually all you can expect to achieve on one wave.

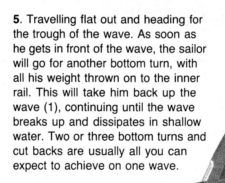

5

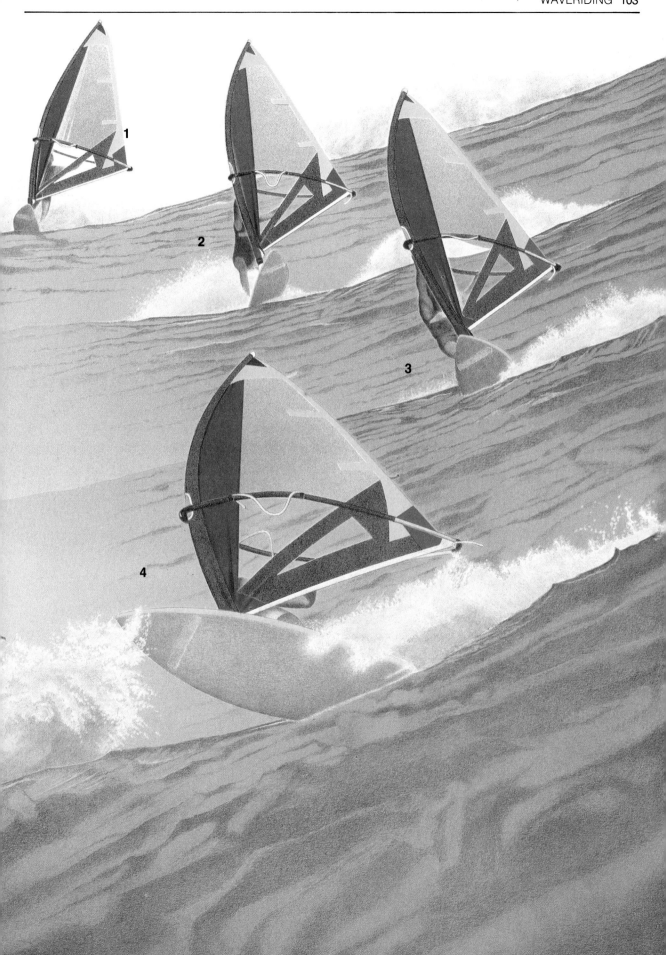

Conditions

The very best conditions for wave riding are found in those places where an open expanse of ocean allows 'ground swell' to develop. Waves are built far out to sea, and when a low pressure storm area occurs the water is driven away from its centre; in the same way you can make a miniature swell by throwing a stone into a pond. As the ocean floor becomes shallow the swell, which has travelled for huge distances, creates waves and when the depth of water can no longer hold these waves they will peak and crumble on the beach.

Sideshore is Best

Waves are also created by localized strong winds, but they usually remain fairly small and can be short lived. The wind direction will determine whether they are good for riding. An onshore wind will tend to make them fold over quickly and become mushy.

Offshore winds hold the waves up longer and this makes classic surfing waves which are, once again, not too good for wind-surfing. Best of all is when the wind is sideshore because this provides a direct line straight out and back through the waves.

Wave Sets

A set of waves occurs when a ground swell is running. Waves tend to come into the beach in periodic sets of three or more.

The first wave in the set is usually the smallest, and the last one the largest. As the set passes it will be much calmer in the area behind the last wave; there is a pause before the next set comes through.

Surfers always look for a set to ride. To spot a set coming, you have to look beyond the break, and you will see a darker area of water – the horizon appears to move up and down much more than usual, which is the sign of an approaching set.

Cut Backs

Cut backs or 'top turns' are used to take you back down the face of the wave towards the steeper, critical section where it's starting to break.
1. The sailor must have enough power and momentum to sail up the wave face.
2. Near the top, but before reaching the lip, weight the inner rail at the tail and sheet in with the rig raked back.
3. You can either make a gradual turn, or a violent slashback style turn, to suit the individual wave.
4. Level the board out, with your weight pushed over the front, to ride down with the wave at maximum speed. When you reach the bottom, get ready to make a bottom turn to take you back up.

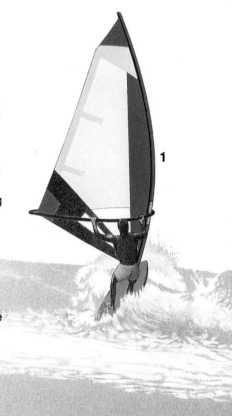

Bottom Turns

This type of turn is made along the bottom of the wave, and is generally used for bearing away along the face. To bottom turn you simply weight the leeward inner rail, and push the rig away from you in the direction you want to go along the wave.
1. Coming down the wave the board travels very fast, so the bottom turn is a real high speed manoeuvre. You go for it just like a gybe – leaning into the turn and weighting the inner rail, but with your back foot remaining in the strap.

The arc of the bottom turn will depend on the wave, and where you want to head back up it to make the most of your ride. With such speed spin-out can be a problem, which is why asymmetric boards with gun style bottom turn sides are favoured in wavesailing locations where the conditions always stay the same.
2. After bottom turning the sailor heads back for the lip. . .
3. . . . and cuts back again.

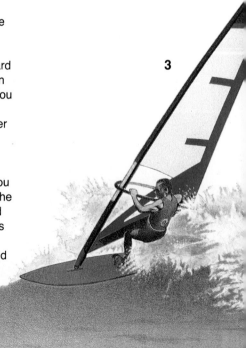

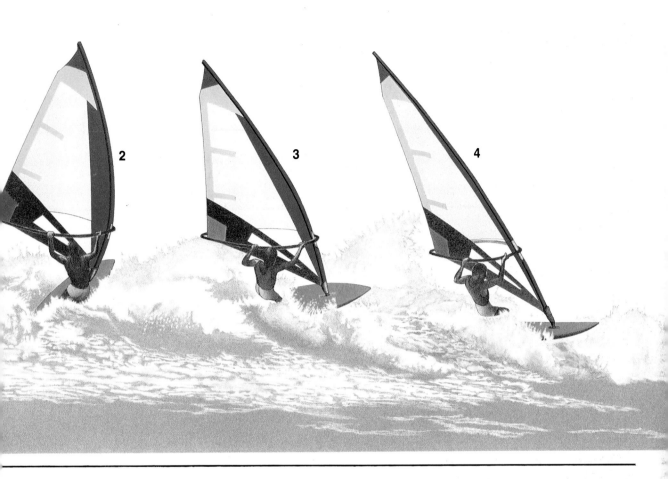

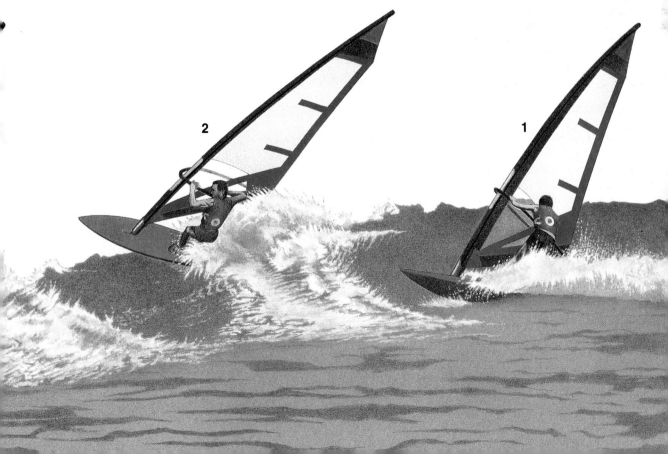

Preparation

You should be really proficient at gybing and waterstarting before sailing waves. Instant changes of direction may be necessary to get out of the path of a fallen sailor or an oncoming wall of white water. Instant waterstarts will also be needed for these same reasons.

Always make sure there are other sailors out there with you, and before launching take a long look at the wave break to work out which are the best areas for jumping and riding. Also find out whether they are affected by tides and currents.

If you're going to be jumping on the way out and riding the waves on the way back in, aim to keep well upwind while jumping so that you have plenty of leeway to ride the waves without ending up a long way downwind.

Equipment

Your equipment will determine the sort of waves you can hope to ride. With sufficient wind and big enough waves, the smaller the board the faster and more manoeuvrable it is likely to be.

The sail should be fully battened or short battened 'soft' style. Make sure then that the boom fits tightly to the mast for a positive connection. Check that there is no way the mastfoot will loosen and come out of the board.

All the components need to be heavy duty, with strength being much more important than light weight. Aluminium, for instance, is no use as it will kink.

You should invest in a special glassfibre 'Wave' mast – some of them are guaranteed against breakage in the surf.

Wave Manoeuvres
Diagram below:
1. Wind direction.
2. Offshore wind holds the wave up for surfing.
3. 'Rip', where water dumped by incoming waves streams back out.
4. Sailing backside along the wave in onshore conditions.
5. Cut back – board is projected back down the wave.
6. Bottom turn to head back up.
7. Easy jumping on the way out in side-onshore winds.
8. Riding backside to the wave.
9. High jump off the steepest part of the wave.
10. Upside-down jump off the steepest part of the wave.
11. Backside bottom turn.
12. Backside off the lip.
13. Frontside bottom turn.
14. Frontside off the lip.

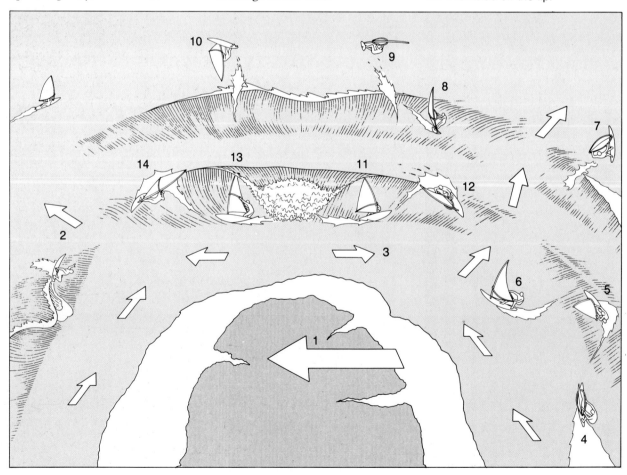

Backside Waveriding

Backside waveriding is usually done in onshore or side-onshore conditions. Once on the wave you have your back to it, with your moves going into the wind, or if it's onshore, parallel with the wind while you stand between the wave and your sail.

To start sailing backside, first luff the board into the wind on the wave face, and then bear away to sail back down it. Don't stall the board too much or the wave may just pass beneath you. A short, highly manoeuvrable board will be able to luff and bear away on the same wave face very quickly; with a longer board it takes more time and is therefore more difficult.

Luffing on to the wave and bearing off down it is done by weighting the inner and outer rails as you would for a gybe.

Luffing and Rollercoasting

This is sometimes called a backside re-entry! It can be performed on any size wave. Luff up to the top as it is starting to break and crumble, and as you hit the top bear away with the white water to travel down and re-enter the wave.

Backside Aerial off the Lip

Great fun on a small, fast board. As you luff up aim to jump off the face at the top of the wave, and then in mid air redirect the board to land back down on the face of white water once again.

Surfing

In light winds catch the wind, bring your front foot forward, and sheet out the rig holding on to it with just one hand to keep the clew out of the water.

You can then use the wave like a surfer, controlling the board by footsteering and balance. See how close you can get the front foot to the nose, preferably 'hanging five' of your toes in classic surfer style.

Lollipop

Bearing off fast along the wave, jump the board as high as possible, aiming to land just in front of the same wave.

Cut Back on White Water

As the wave begins to close over into white water, hit it in the critical section and bear radically away from the wind.

Below: Riding backside on an Atlantic roller. Frontside waveriding is more demanding, but has greater potential for radical manoeuvres.

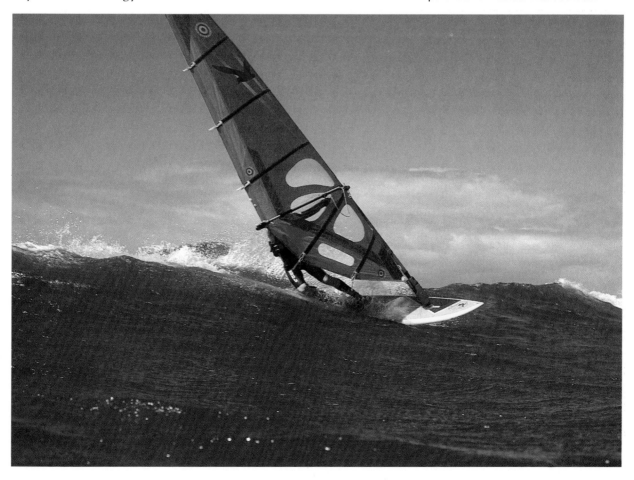

Frontside Waveriding

Frontside wave conditions occur when you can bear away for the wave face, with the sail between your body and the wave.

Most Hawaiian waveriding is frontside, and you need sideshore or side-offshore winds (as they have there) to allow you to bear off on to the wave. Frontside conditions are only found where there is a good ground swell running, as the offshore wind will have the effect of flattening smaller, wind blown waves.

S-Turning

Frontside waveriding is more difficult than backside, because it's harder to see what the wave is doing. This makes timing and judgement highly important. When you first try going frontside, catch the swell and practise bearing away and then slowly bringing the board back on its original course.

This is called *S-Turning*, and it's difficult to learn because when you bear away and up the face, your board is liable to stall. The nose must be kept well up so that it cannot dig into the wave, and the critical breaking section should be avoided by cutting back and luffing back down the face.

Off the Lip

This is not necessarily as radical a manoeuvre as it sounds. It can be performed on a huge wave with the board exploding off the top. Or it can be done more easily and slowly on a small wave, when it's just a progression of the cut back. The difference is that you head the board straight for the lip, and then cut back with a major shift of direction in the instant when you hit the lip.

Rollercoaster

This is when you hit the critical breaking section of the wave, and rollercoast down on to the crumbling wave's white water.

Off the Lip

An off the lip is a radical variation on a cut back where the sailor actually hits the breaking lip of the wave, before projecting his board back down amidst the churning, white water. Timing is critical, or an unpleasant wipe-out will be the result. This illustration shows how to go for it at full power.
1. Having gone for a maximum speed bottom turn, the sailor powers himself up towards the lip aiming at a point which is still unbroken.
2. He carves round to hit the lip at a gravity defying angle, pushing the board up to it by straightening his legs with his weight hung back over the tail and ready to pivot on it.
3. All his weight is taken by the boom as the wave pushes the nose of the board round for the ride back down in the crumbling white water.

Aerial Off the Lip

Similar to an off the lip, but much more tricky. When you hit the lip your board must be directed on and up into the air, before landing back on the wave further down the line.
1. First a high speed run up towards the lip with all the momentum from the bottom turn.
2. He hits it at maximum speed, before projecting the board straight on up into the air.
3. As the tail leaves the lip he pushes out the tail to redirect the board so that it lands back on the face and heads down the wave.

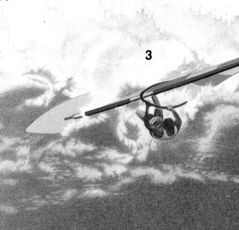

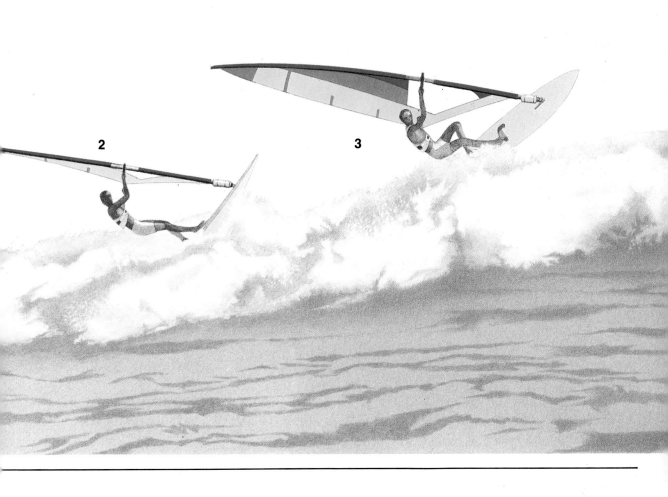

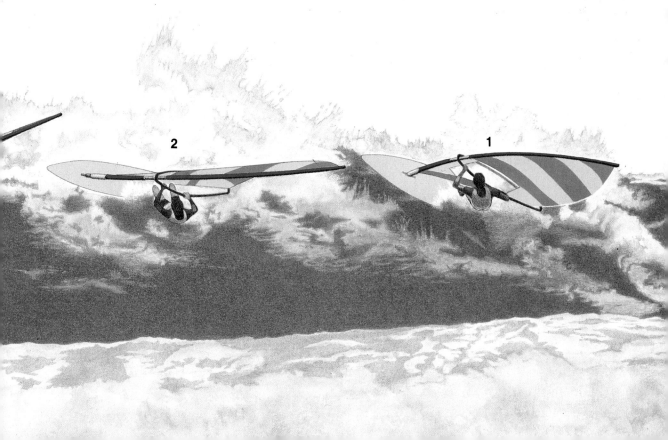

Accidents Happen

All windsurfers are bound to take a fall sometimes, and it is important to know how to handle it properly.

The first essential is that you should never get in front of the board and rig with the wave behind it. If this does happen, the best action is to dive underwater to one side to put yourself well clear of it all.

You should always try to keep with the rig and the board. They are your only means of flotation, and if you lose them you will have to swim which can be unnerving and tiring in big surf.

You should try to stay relaxed. Waves will take you in towards the beach anyway and you can use this to your advantage. Small ones can be body surfed by swimming hard just before they reach you; with bigger ones you will need to dive underwater for a few seconds to let each one pass by and avoid being pummelled.

The easiest way to keep yourself together with both board and rig is to swim the mast tip into the waves. As each wave comes you will have to push the tip as far underwater as possible, and then just hang on.

Wipe Out!

Big waves can be dangerous, and when there are needle nosed boards flying around at well over 40 knots it is doubly hazardous.

There are plenty of grisly surfing tales of surfers being impaled and even decapitated by their boards. Luckily windsurfing seems less accident prone, though when short board sailing you must pay constant attention to safety.

This is a matter of being able to handle your board, and knowing the rights of way. Before going out in the waves, you must be sure that you can cope with the conditions, or you will be a liability to everyone else whether they are windsurfing or surfing.

Rights of Way

Collisions on waves can be very dangerous, and should never happen. You must understand and abide by the basic rights-of-way rules. Unfortunately you can't be sure that everybody else out there will know what they're up to, so look out for idiots and be prepared to be tolerant and take avoiding action when necessary.

The rules for waveriding are no more than a variation on those for all windsurfing:

Boards on the same tack:
★ Starboard (when you're standing on the right hand side of the board) has right of way over port tack.

Boards on different tacks:
★ The overtaking board keeps clear.
★ The board which is pointing higher has right of way over the one which is pointing lower when they converge.

For waveriding in surf conditions you must remember:
★ Windsurfers always give way to surfers (and swimmers if there are any around).
★ The first sailor on a wave has rights to ride that wave over any other sailor.
★ If two sailors catch the same wave at the same time, the one who is upwind has right of way.
★ Sailors who are changing course or gybing have no right of way.
★ Sailors waterstarting must wait until they have a clear path to get going.

Other points worth noting:
★ Always look before you change course. If you want to go into a fast gybe, look through the window to check that no one is in your path downwind. A lot of accidents are caused this way, and it's not much fun for the other guy when the nose of your board drives into his back at 30 knots.
★ If a collision seems inevitable and you reckon you have right of way, let the other guy know – just yell!

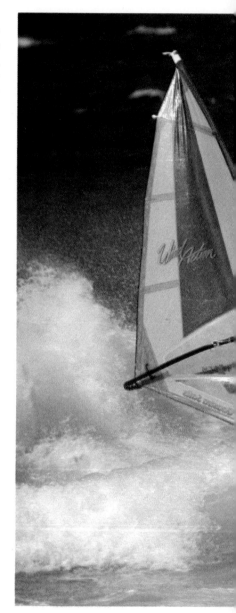

Injuries

In wavesailing the body can be pushed beyond its normal limits, since some of the contortions required are closer to gymnastics than ordinary windsurfing.

Muscle, ligament and bone injuries are sometimes the result. To guard against them:
1. Do regular stretching and strengthening exercises so that you are fit to sail.
2. Do warm-up exercises on the

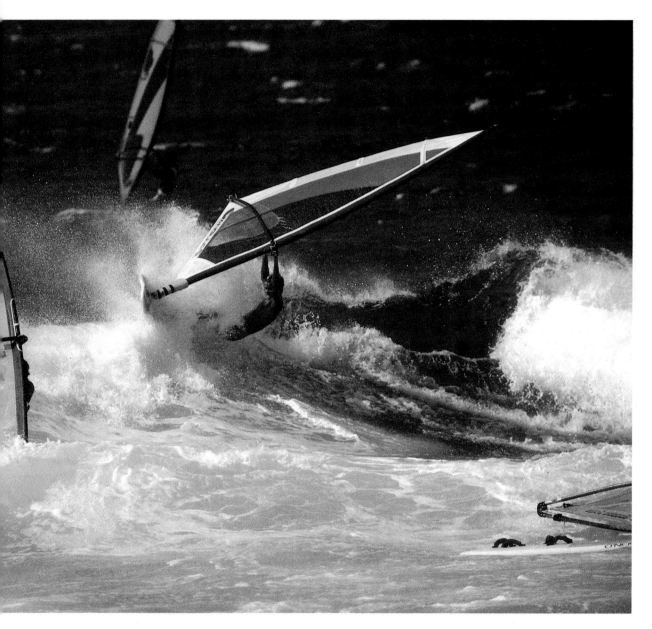

beach before wavesailing.

In addition every sailor should know basic first aid so that he can be of assistance in emergencies. If you are unfortunate enough to be injured and are unable to get back to the shore, try and stay on your board and attract attention by shouting and yelling for help.

Severe Cold

Cold wind and water can result in hypothermia which first shows itself by loss of muscle co-ordination, lack of clear thinking, and general fatigue and drowsiness. If it is left to get worse hypothermia can eventually result in death, so if you have any of the symptoms you should head back for the shore.

If you are unable to get back your priority should be to maintain body temperature. Get up on the board if it will support your weight, and do warm-up exercises with as much of your body out of

Above: Accidents happen! When you're out in the waves be sure you can handle the conditions and always stick to the rights-of-way rules.

the water as possible. If you are unable to stay on the board, don't thrash around in the water as this will make you lose body heat – just huddle up and wait for rescue.

Immediately you are back on shore dry yourself and wrap up as warmly as possible.

Competition

Sailing a short board is competition in itself – competition against the waves and the wind, and a challenge to master increasingly radical techniques with more and more radical equipment.

However, there may come a time when it's nice to measure your speed against others out on the water, and to establish just how advanced you are at short board handling. If you have reached this stage yourself you can choose from three different types of competition, as described below.

Slalom

This is the most popular kind of short board racing; it evolved from the ins-and-outs held during the Pan Am Cup in Hawaii (now sadly a thing of the past). It is an equal test of short board handling and speed with short reaching legs, numerous gybes, and frequently difficult conditions in the breaking surf near the shoreline.

Wave Performance

This is a test of wave sailing ability which relies heavily on good waveriding conditions. It is purely a test of the riders' skill in sailing on waves. It is marked by a panel of judges in a very similar way to a sport like freestyle ice skating.

Speed Trials

This is solely a test of speed, held over a 500 metre course. There are half a dozen major international events in the calendar, and from among them are usually a new World Speed Record, sometimes more than once a year. Windsurfers are now officially recognized as the fastest sailing craft in the world.

Right: David Daly going through his routine during the O'Neill Invitational at Hookipa. This is one of the major wave performance events in the international calendar and it takes place in the spring of each year.

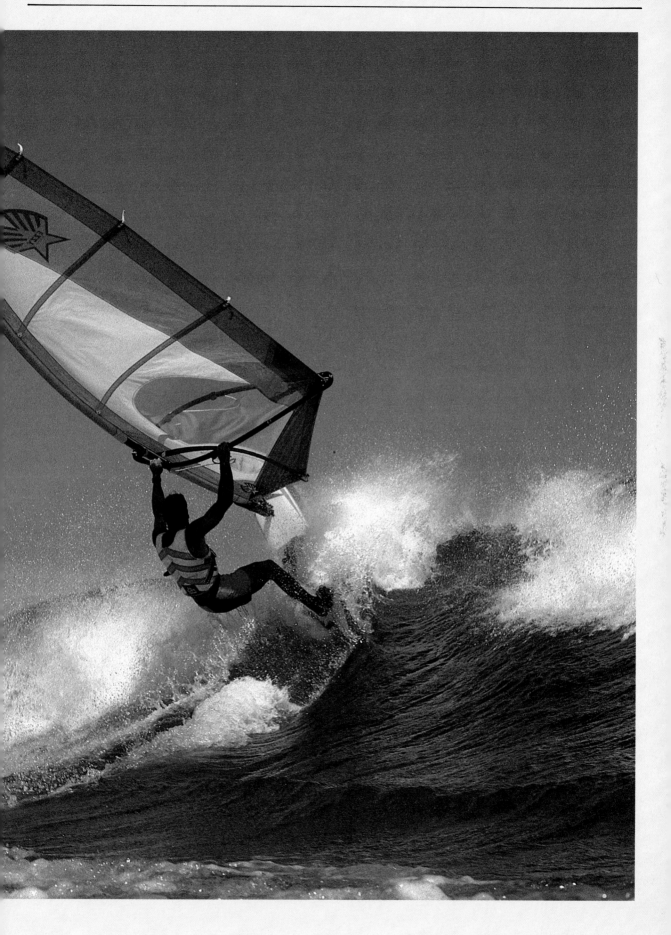

Slalom

Slalom races are most easily and effectively started from the beach. This is because the boards almost always need to be waterstarted which precludes laying a conventional start line on the water.

The most suitable course is usually the figure of eight as shown in the diagram below.

The World Cup norm is for eight competitors to race in each heat, with a maximum of the first four sailors going through to the next heat and working on towards the final.

Rules are Vital

Right of way rules are very important, not least because there is a very real risk of injury if competitors collide. Remember, the combined speeds in a head-on crash can be as much as 50 knots! The World Cup rules are a good basis for any slalom competition:

1. A competitor coming in (with the waves) shall keep clear of a competitor going out (against the waves).
2. A competitor clean astern shall keep clear of a competitor clear ahead when on the same tack or gybing.

3. An overtaking competitor shall keep clear.
4. A competitor who is sailing shall avoid a competitor who has fallen off.
5. A competitor who is waterstarting after a fall shall keep clear of all competitors who are sailing.

Equipment

Boards used will depend on the wind speed, but if racing with the World Cup recommended minimum of 11 knots they will be fairly small.

As an example Robby Naish, who was World Cup Slalom Champion from 1983–1986 used two boards during the 1986 season for light (Force 4–5) and strong (Force 5–6 and above) conditions. Both featured the same simple rounded pintail outline, with a single concave nose leading to double concave mid sections.

Both boards were around 2.70 m (8 ft 10 in) long with 33 cm (13 in) maximum width. The main difference was that the lighter wind version was made thicker for more volume. All slalom boards have a single fin to maximize speed.

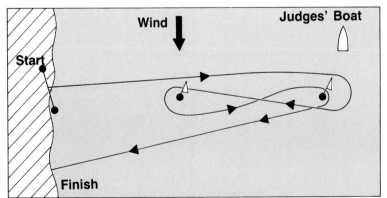

Slalom Course

The figure of eight slalom course is ideally set so that it takes competitors in and out through breaking surf, making it a really tough test of short board handling. Distance between the marks is usually 400–800 metres, competitors going round as many as five times.

The Start

Rule number one is avoid thy neighbour – and don't let him crowd you. If you've had the luck to draw a windward or leeward starting position, you have some latitude for getting away – if you're to windward, run to windward; if you're to leeward, run to leeward.

Decide when sailing is going to be faster than running. Many sailors jump on their board too

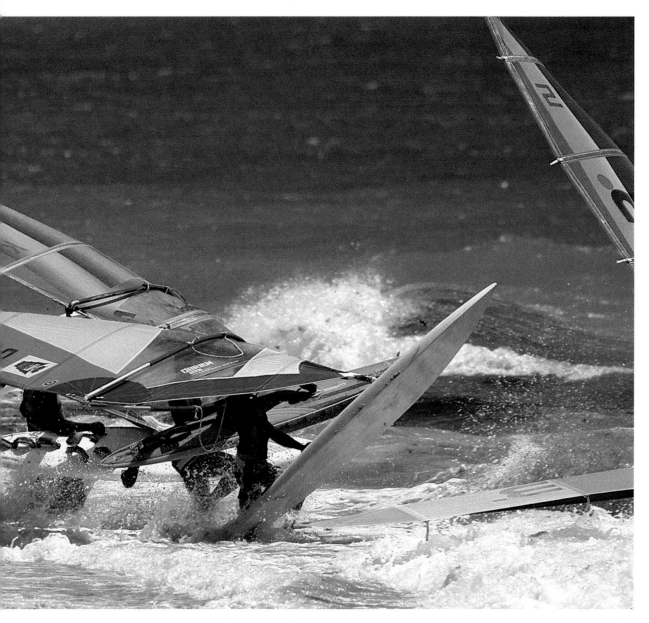

early, letting others run into the water and start well ahead.

The Reaches

You should reach up to the marks at maximum speed. If the distance is short, the course is high, your board doesn't point well, and you're crowded you will need to work to windward before you can attack those who are ahead.

If, however, you can fetch the marks with no problem, you should bear away for top speed and clean air, and go all out to get ahead.

The Mark Roundings

Rounding the mark will depend on your gybing skill – if you only know the smooth, sweeping arc style of gybe you will have to allow space to windward. If you can do tight gybes, you will be able to suit your position to the conditions and other competitors.

Above: A slalom start – just pick up your board and run into the water, try to keep clear of the confusion on all sides. A quick getaway is vital.

If waves are making the rounding difficult, slowing down and waiting for the right moment will almost certainly be faster than going all out for it and falling.

It's consistency, skill, and a little bit of luck for the sailor which wins slalom races.

Wave Performance

Wave performance competitions are equally good for participants and spectators, because it involves man-on-man competition with each sailor trying to outdo the other in good view of the beach!

If, for instance, there are 70 entrants, they are divided into pairs. The first round is usually run with two pairs in each heat, with heats of up to eight minutes long. (Final round are usually of from 12–15 minutes.)

The two winners in the first round go through to the *winners'* side, and the two losers to the *losers'* side; eventually the winner of the *winners* meets the winner of the *losers* in a best-of-three final. This double elimination sounds complicated, but it gives each competitor two chances to progress to the next round, while he has only one if the event is run as a sudden death single elimination.

The Judges

There can be three or five judges; they have a view of the competition area which is delineated by two large marker buoys. If a competitor leaves the area his performance is not scored.

The judges mark the three disci-

Bottom left: Man-on-man! One sailor bottom turns on the inside to ride up the wave, while the other kicks out in a jump for maximum height and style. Both are trying to collect points before the final hooter tells them that their heat is over.

Bottom right: This is Mark Angulo in action during a wave event at Hookipa. A radical manoeuvre like this will score maximum points, but you have to find the right compromise between impressing the judges and staying up on your board. If you wipe out 40 per cent of the time, you're unlikely to win.

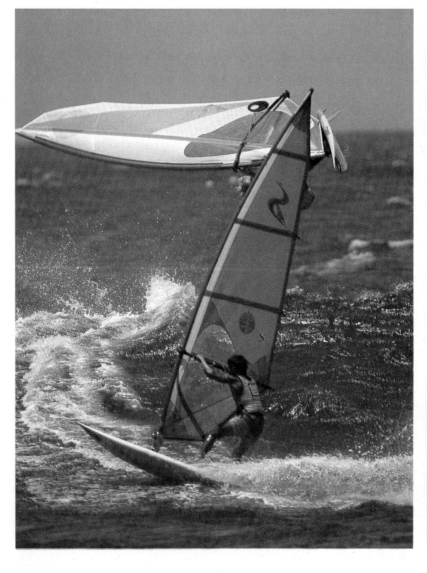

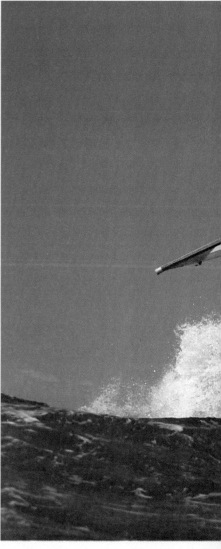

plines of wave performance according to style and difficulty:
1. Wave riding.
2. Wave jumping.
3. Transitions.

The marking system has no set form, but most use a scale of one to ten within each category, these marks are totalled to reach the score for that heat.

The judges also check that the competitors conform to the wave performance rules, which are summarized in 'Accidents Happen' on page 110. They are there for your safety and are a development of the right of way rules.

Conditions

Most world class events are held in Hawaii and Australia, where conditions are consistent – reef breaks and Trade Winds supply the necessary waves and average 13 knot winds.

Local conditions dictate the type of routine you go for to impress the judges. High winds and big waves allow more riding and jumping; lighter winds and small waves call for more flashy transitional manoeuvres.

What you have to do is draw upon your reserve of tricks and manoeuvres, and complete as

many as possible during the allocated time. You must, however, be confident of performing each one successfully – falls are just valuable time wasted in the water.

The hooter goes when there are two minutes to the start of your heat. You then have the choice of beginning your routine on the 'outside' and riding in, or on the 'inside' by jumping out. After that it's a succession of working the waves, making the necessary transitions with plenty of style variations (one handed duck gybes etc), and jumping for maximum height and appearance.

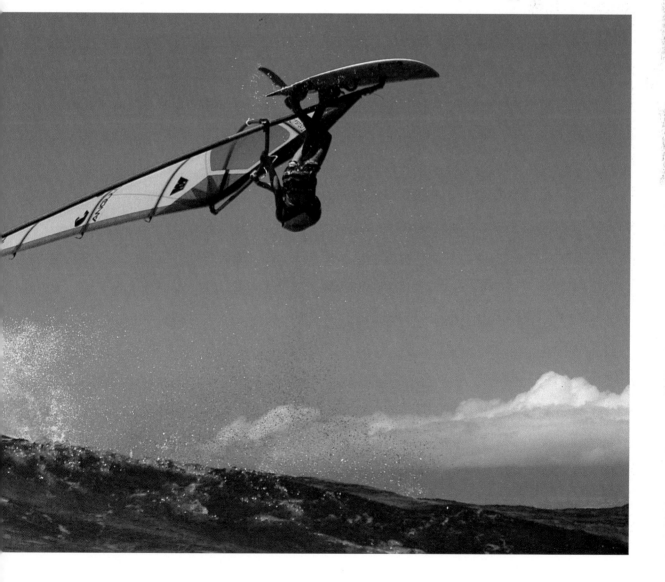

Speed Trials

The quest for speed is in some ways the most fascinating of short board competitions, and is a clear reflection of the enormous advances which have been made in windsurfing in a comparatively short time.

In 1977 Derk Thijs of the Netherlands recorded 17.1 knots over a 500 metre course during Weymouth Speed Week. He was sailing a specially light Windglider, and his speed was regarded as amazing. In July 1986 (almost nine years later) Pascal Maka bumped the record up to 38.86 knots over the same 500 metres at a speed event held in Fuerteventura – well over twice the speed!

In between there were many records, with the speeds increasing in line with new designs and materials.

Venues

The longest-running and most highly regarded speed event is Weymouth Speed Week, held in Britain's Portland Harbour in October. This venue combines the classic speed trial requirements of very high winds with water that is as flat as possible.

The high winds are brought in by the Atlantic equinoctial gales which are accelerated up, over and down the enormous shingle bank of Chesil Beach before swooping over the broad expanse of Portland Harbour.

Speed sailors make their runs close to the shore, receiving the full blast of the wind at around shoulder height, while the surface water remains relatively calm.

Portland has claimed more records than any other venue (Derk Thijs, 1977; Clive Colenso, 1979; Pascal Maka, 1982; Fred Haywood, 1983).

Setting a Record

For a new record to be ratified, the event must be observed by the RYA. The new record must be at least two per cent faster than the previous time to allow for any slight discrepancy in timing.

This procedure established new records at Port St Louis in the south of France in 1985 (Michael Pucher), and in Sotavento on the southern tip of Fuerteventura in 1986 (Pascal Maka). Other venues where conditions seem conducive to record breaking include the 'Ponds' in California, near Los Angeles, and Lethbridge near Alberta. Even when records are not set, there is usually a handsome prize for each speed event's winner and the international speed circuit is well patronized.

Equipment

Contemporary speed sailors favour relatively simple, very small guns, with single or double concave V tail bottoms. The chosen length is usually 2.30–2.50 m (7 ft 6 in – 8 ft 2 in), and most boards are so narrow – around 30 cm (12 in) max – that it is really like sailing on an over-grown waterski!

In recent times the most popular designer has been Jimmy Lewis of Maui, who has shaped boards for most of the top names. Like most speed boards, his are of conventional custom construction.

Fred Haywood broke the record in 1983 with the first 'wing' rig, and since then there has been much work concentrated on sail design. Most recently the multi batten camber induced variety have ruled the scene. They are used in conjunction with super stiff pre-bent masts, sometimes with aluminium battens for the ultimate ratio of stiffness to weight.

Speed Technique

The optimum wind direction for a speed course is reckoned to be around 140 degrees, which gives a very broad reach. This enables the sailor to handle a big sail in powerful winds, without the

board being blown too much sideways (as would happen on a closer reach).

For a time it was assumed that speed sailors needed to be huge men sailing in the strongest winds.

Recently, however, it's become apparent that lightweight sailors with small sails can go just as fast as a heavyweight with a big sail in the same wind conditions.

Apart from handling the sail, the

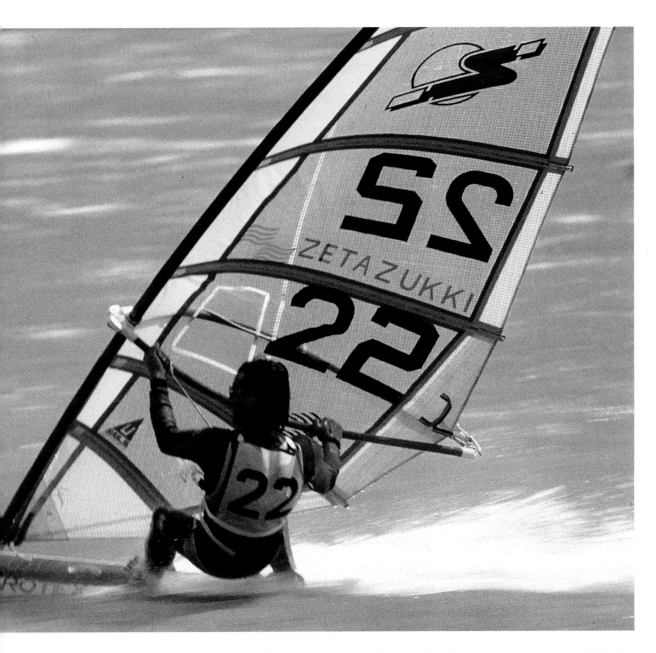

principal skill in speedsailing is to complete the course without spinning out. This is a matter of keeping the skeg in the water when the board hits chop, using your legs as shock absorbers to soak up the impact; or if necessary pre-jumping the chop in the style of speed skiers.

The Speed Sailors

Top class speed sailors train hard to achieve the kind of control necessary for high speed records. It's interesting to note that the fastest four sailors at the record making 1986 Fuerteventura speed event – Pascal Maka, Eric Beale, Jimmy Lewis and Fred Haywood – had spent the previous spring training together on Maui, all using Jimmy Lewis to design and make their boards.

Their speeds ranged from 36.13

Above: Peter Bridgman (UK), one of the seasoned campaigners on the world's speed circuit. He designs and makes his own boards in Venice.

knots up to Maka's 38.36 knot record. This made them the only sailors who had ever gone faster than the previous 36 knot outright world speed sailing record. This was established in 1979 by the 60 foot British proa *Crossbow*.

Speedsailing

What do you do when there's not enough wind? Answer: If you have a nice expanse of hard sandy beach, go speedsailing.

The speedsail was invented by Baron Arnaud de Rosnay, and in essence it's an elongated skateboard with a windsurfer rig mounted on it. There are a number of refinements such as a wider base, larger blow-up wheels, and trucks which can withstand heavy use in a salt water location; but the basic principles of a skateboard are there, plus the advantage of having a rig to power you.

The speedsail is carved right or left by weighting it just like a short board. However, the lack of friction between its wheels and a hard surface makes it far faster than any board, and speeds of up to 50 mph come comparatively easily – this explains the crash hats and heavy duty protection used.

The great thing about a speedsail is that you can use it to practise and work out all your short board manoeuvres on dry land. Carve gybes, duck gybes and 360's are all normal fare for speedsails. As long as you have enough nerve not to worry about falling, they are much easier to perform with a speedsail because it will just keep rolling on, whereas a board would be stalling.

What's Available?

There are a number of varieties of speedsail, but the original version which is still one of the best is the Norbert Blanc Speed Sail which is manufactured in France.

This is the speedsail shown in the photo, and all you need to add to make it go is your short board rig – a sail around five sq m (54 sq ft) is the maximum you'll need without risking a kamikaze act.

Right: Flat out at over 40 mph on a close reach during the third Speed Sail World Championships. This event was held on Saunton Sands, in North Devon, England.

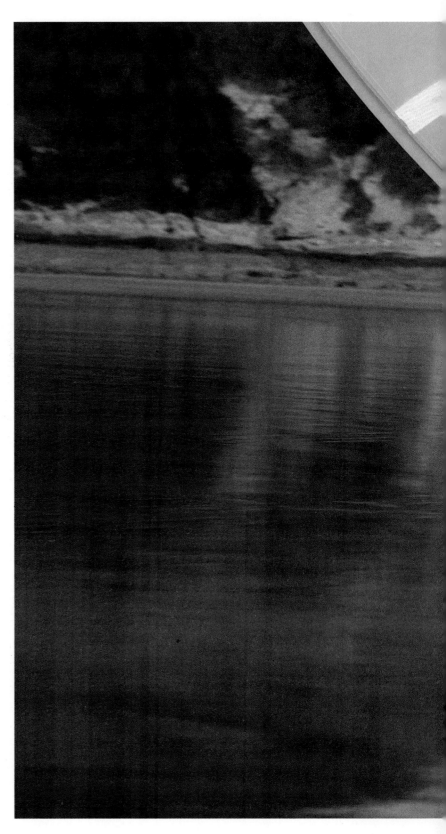

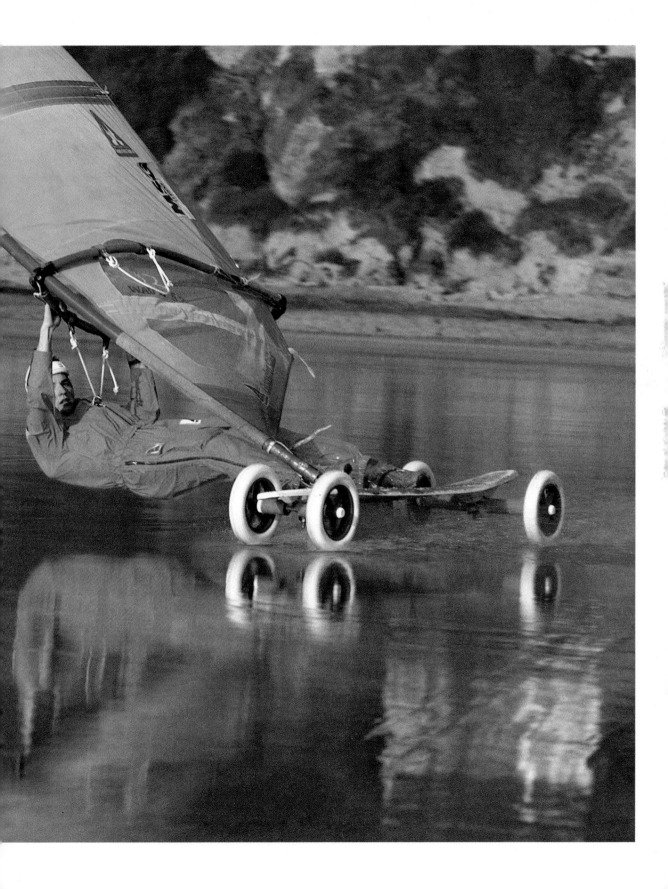

Repairs

Short boards are susceptible to damage, particularly custom models which, although strong when on the water, are very fragile when they are on the land.

The lesson is to always carry the board when it's not on the water, but this is not always as easy as it sounds. Boards are washed on to pebbly beaches in a shorebreak and can be blown off roofracks, and some kind of impact damage is bound to result. If this is minor, simple repairs can be made with an epoxy adhesive such as *Araldite*, though you should check with the maker that this is suitable for your particular board.

1. *Before starting work*: The repair area must be clean, de-greased and dry; instructions and mixing ratios must be understood; ventilation and the possibility of fire must be allowed for; ambient working temperature must be at least 20°C.

If there is foam damage, cut away the skin to clean material, and then dig out any wet or soft foam with a knife. A small hole can be filled with epoxy resin or Araldite; if it's a large hole the heat build-up from the resin may melt the surrounding foam, so you will have to fill it with PU foam.

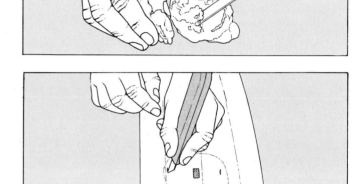

2. Make the hole perfect with no sharp edges, and then roughen the surrounding skin using sandpaper. Cover the repair area with strips of adhesive masking tape, and use a knife to cut a central hole through which you can pour the foam, plus smaller air holes round the sides.

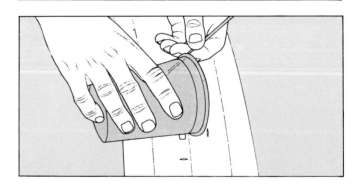

3. Mix the two components of the PU foam. Depending on the mixture and the air temperature, the liquid will begin to expand and solidify fairly quickly. Pour it through the central hole in the tape, and tape this over. You should be able to calculate roughly how much foam is required, but excess will escape through the small air holes. PU foam must be used whether the core is PU or polystyrene. The two foams are compatible, but only PU is available as a liquid.

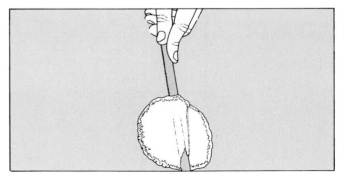

4. After the specified hardening time the tape can be removed. The brown PU foam will have risen in a bump, so cut off the excess above the skin with a hacksaw blade. Then sandpaper the foam until it is level with the underside of the skin.

More Extensive DIY

Slightly larger repairs are not too difficult for those who have an inclination for DIY. Glassfibre can be used to replace an area of broken skin and the foam beneath can be replaced with polyurethane foam. The work demands a fair amount of care and patience, so if you're in doubt it might be better to use a specialist repair service.

Apart from impact damage it's possible to break out skeg boxes, weaken mast boxes and dent the foam behind the footstraps under your heels. All this damage can usually be repaired by replacing the damaged material.

5. Use the hacksaw blade or a knife to make a 5 mm (3/16 in) deep horizontal cut all around the perimeter of the hole beneath the skin. This will ensure that the replacement skin has a good bond to both foam and skin.

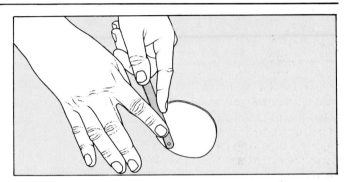

6. Mask around the repair area, and use a brush to stipple epoxy resin on the foam up to the edges. Drop on chopped strand mat glassfibre, keeping it wet with the resin and building up the depth until you can tuck the glassfibre into the 5 mm slit, using the knife or hacksaw blade. Continue building up the depth of the glassfibre, until it is level with or slightly above the other skin.

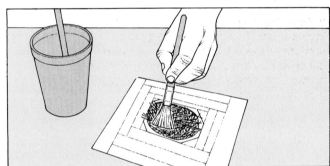

7. When the glassfibre has completely cured (follow instructions carefully) remove the tape. Sandpaper the glassfibre until it is approximately 1 mm (1/32 in) below the level of the outer skin. Then apply a polyester filler such as Plastic Padding. When this has hardened, file it down to the top surface taking care not to damage the surrounding area, and then use wet and dry sandpaper until it is smooth and flush with the outer skin. For the best possible finish apply another layer made up of cellulose car body putty, and rub it down with fine grade wet and dry.

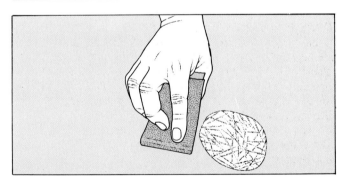

8. You can then paint the repair area with brush or spray gun. The latter gives a much better finish. Use acrylic paint, or special non-slip paint if it's on the deck area.

This epoxy repair technique can be modified and adapted for most short board damage. However some moulded board manufacturers specify particular materials for repairs, so you should contact them if you have any doubts.

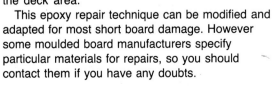

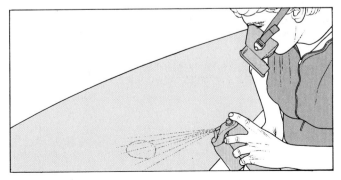

Top Places

There are many good places for short board sailing, and it would be impossible to cover them all. This section concentrates on four major areas which can be recommended to any enthusiast – Hawaii, the Canary Islands, the Columbia Gorge, and the UK's West Country.

Other locations may be as good, if not better. Depending on where and when you want to travel, there are a number of places you could add to the list of choices.

The Caribbean

The Caribbean islands benefit from hot sun, palm trees, lots of rum, and Trade Winds. Most of the islands are fine for long boards, but the winds may be a little marginal for short boards. One of the exceptions is Barbados which has perfect sideshore winds around its south-western tip. It offers excellent conditions for those who want to learn or improve their short board sailing at Oistins Bay, and even better conditions for those who are real hot shots off the big reef break at Silver Sands. Both spots have Club Mistral facilities.

The Western Mediterranean

Tarifa is on the southern tip of Spain, near the point where the Mediterranean becomes the Atlantic. The narrow straits which divide it from North Africa help to create two winds – the Poniente which blows Force 3–6 from the west; and the Levante which blows Force 6–8 from the east. Conditions are usually wind blown chop; the weather is hot in summer; and there's a Club Mistral.

Further east, the north of Sardinia by the Straits of Bonifacio is another area which had good reliable short board winds. Porto Pollo is the main centre, with a F2 Club on hand.

The Eastern Mediterranean

The islands of the Greek Aegean are noted for strong thermal winds in the summer, which exceed Force 4 on most afternoons. No waves, but plenty of wind blown chop, and of course Greece is a very cheap country for living and eating. The best known islands for short board sailing are Kos, Milos, and Paros. Nearby, the coast of Turkey also has the same thermal conditions.

Right: After a hard day's sailing just pack up your gear and drive the jeep home, ready for another hard day's sailing the next day. This is the life on Fuerteventura in the Canary Islands.

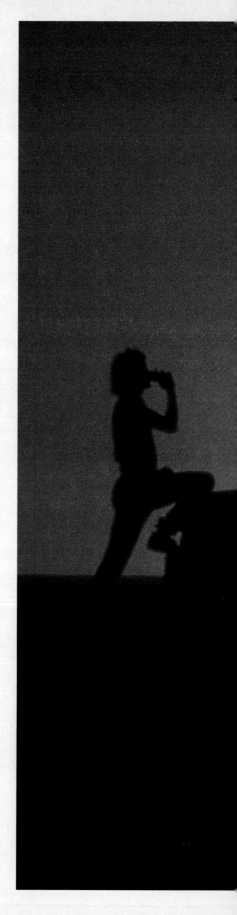

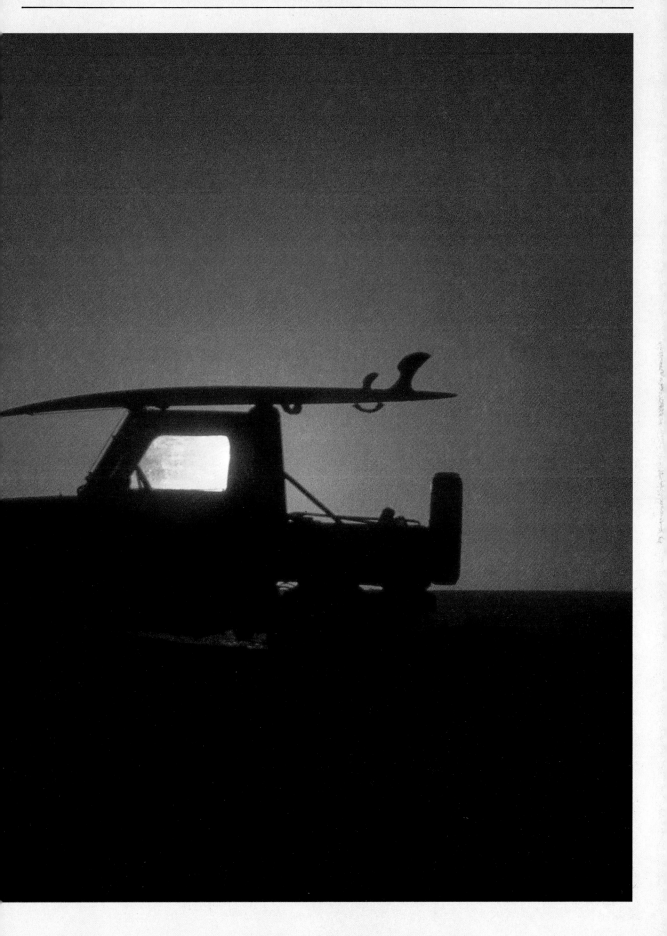

Hawaii

Ever since windsurfing first began, Hawaii has been recognized as the mecca of the sport – and it has grown and developed over the years from the old Windsurfer Rocket days to the current high performance boards and sails.

Hawaii has this high status because of its warm climate, consistent Trade Winds, and perfect waves which are ideal for putting all the latest equipment to the test.

However, despite the general impression of huge waves and wind every day, there are many white, sandy beaches with few waves and where winds blow at no more than 10–20 knots. With year round air temperatures between 65–88°F and average water temperatures of 76°F, Hawaii is excellent for all kinds of windsurfing holidays.

Eight Islands

Hawaii is made up of eight main islands plus quite a few smaller ones. Seven are populated, with Oahu being the capital island.

All the Hawaiian islands offer variations of what Oahu provides for the windsurfer, but the outer islands, being further afield and less accessible, tend to be more expensive to use as sailing venues.

Oahu

As you come in to land you will see the Honolulu skyscrapers – it's just like any other international city, and you won't see anything like it in the rest of Hawaii.

The tourist area is Waikiki and that's where most of the (fairly expensive) hotels are located. Getting around the island is easiest by car, but it's unfortunate that the area has a bad reputation for car break-ins.

Windsurfing on Oahu is a major sport, and equipment is widely available for hire to short board enthusiasts in both Waikiki and Kailua – in the latter you can visit the famous emporiums of Windsurfing Hawaii and Naish Hawaii.

In the prevailing Trade Wind conditions the windward Kailua side will have more onshore winds, while the leeward Waikiki/ Diamond Head side is more offshore. With shelter from a reef Kailua offers basically fairly flat water with steady winds up to half a mile (800 m) out, while there are bigger swells and more wind in the deep water further out to sea.

The famous Diamond Head is one of the world's leading wavesailing locations, and is shallow enough for you to scrape your feet on the sharp coral at low tide. It's best in spring and summer when the southerly swells can rise as high as 15 feet (4.50 m) with wind coming from the east daily. The biggest problem there is the

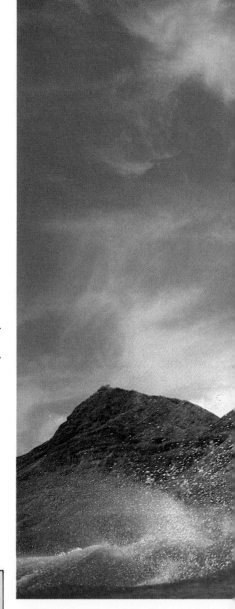

Above: Randy Naish blasts off from Diamond Head. If you can't waterstart or gybe well don't attempt to sail here – the coral is very unforgiving.
Left: The principal islands of the Hawaiian chain. They tend to become quieter the further you are away from Oahu which is the main centre. The island of Hawaii is called 'The Big Island', much of which is inaccessible.

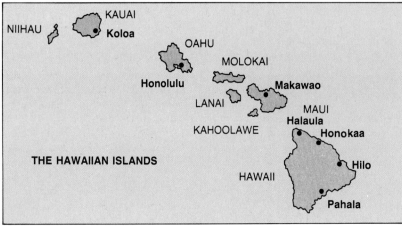

THE HAWAIIAN ISLANDS

NIIHAU
KAUAI
Koloa
OAHU
Honolulu
MOLOKAI
Makawao
LANAI
MAUI
KAHOOLAWE
Halaula
Honokaa
Hilo
HAWAII
Pahala

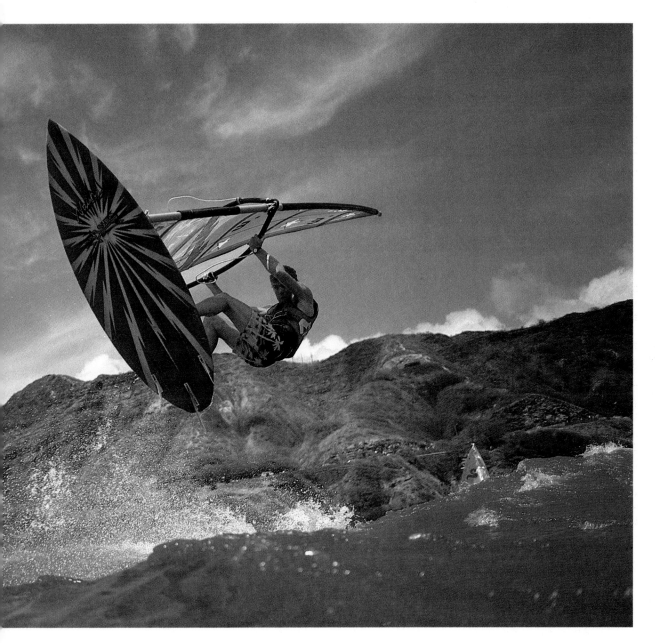

long hike with all your gear from the car down to the beach.

Backyards on the North Shore is the most advanced place to sail on Oahu, and is located near to the Pipeline and Sunset surf beaches. It is only suitable for absolute experts who are willing to try windsurfing in waves twice mast height.

Maui

Maui is much quieter than Oahu, and it's the home of Hookipa where both the Maui Grand Prix and O'Neill Wave Classic take place each year. It's about a 30 minute flight from Honolulu, and if the North Shore style swells of Hookipa are too much for you (most radical during the winter months), less extreme conditions can be found at Sprecklesville and S-Turns. Many famous windsurfers make Maui their home.

Kauai, Hawaii, Molokai

These three islands all have lesser known spots where you will find seclusion and excellent conditions, though access to some of the launch sites can be difficult.

For all the Hawaiian islands, the best time for wind, weather and cost is the summer. The winds blow 10–20 knots from the east-north-east virtually every day, but are much more variable in winter.

The Canaries

Sited in the Atlantic off the North African coastline, the Canary Islands are rated as the number one winter windsurfing location for all of Europe's short board sailors.

The climate during their winter is comparatively mild, with an average 68°F mid-day temperature in January which is the coldest month. The sea temperature at this time is dropping towards its low point of 64°F which makes a steamer style wetsuit a necessity. In summer the water warms up to around 72°F and average daytime temperatures peak around 90°F.

Trade Wind Conditions

The principal winds are the northeast Trades, but as in Hawaii these are much more consistent during the summer, when they are also bolstered by the thermal effect of the sun. Between May and September you would be unlucky not to experience good short board winds on most days; but during the winter the winds are much more fitful, and can be light or very strong depending on the Atlantic depressions.

The amount of wind at any one time can vary enormously, it depends on where you are. There are local variations – such as the wind funnelling between the islands or sweeping down the steep mountain sides.

Fuerteventura

Fuerteventura's sand dunes attract sun worshippers in all states of undress, and its sailing conditions attract wavesailors who rate it as the best spot on the east side of the Atlantic.

Having a car is essential, and as with all the islands car rental is readily available and reasonably cheap. The principal spots are:

Cotillo

A mile long sandy beach facing west, and picking up big swells from the Atlantic. The steep, shelving beach makes big, hollow waves which tend to close out, and during the winter they can be pretty powerful.

Shooting Gallery

Half a mile to the west of Corralejo (the island's windsurfing capital), the Shooting Gallery pushes up excellent high performance waves that are reckoned to rival any break in Hawaii. Launching is difficult because of the reef, and waves can be mast high. They are sideshore.

Harbour Wall

The outside of Corralejo's harbour wall offers similar conditions to the Shooting Gallery but with smaller waves.

Corralejo Bay/The Point

Conditions vary from flat water to waves, and are likely to be forgiving for the less expert short board sailor. As with most of the launch spots, the area is ringed with sharp volcanic rock.

Flag Beach/Ulli's Beach

Down the east coast the beaches become progressively more sandy and user friendly, but you will only find swell after a Scirocco.

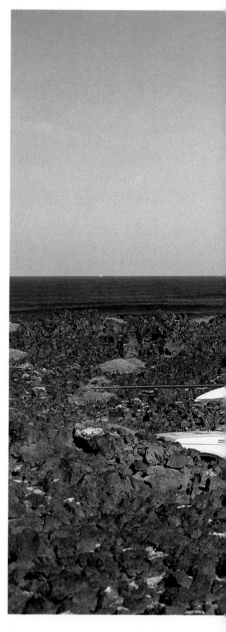

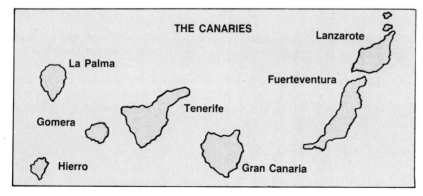

THE CANARIES

La Palma

Lanzarote

Fuerteventura

Tenerife

Gomera

Hierro

Gran Canaria

Above: The north coast of Fuerteventura near the Shooting Gallery (named after a nearby clay pigeon range). Fuerteventura is rated the best of the Canaries.

Left: The north-east Trade Winds funnel between the islands. The long, slim outline of Fuerteventura is angled to take most advantage of these winds, and boasts many more sailing spots than the other islands.

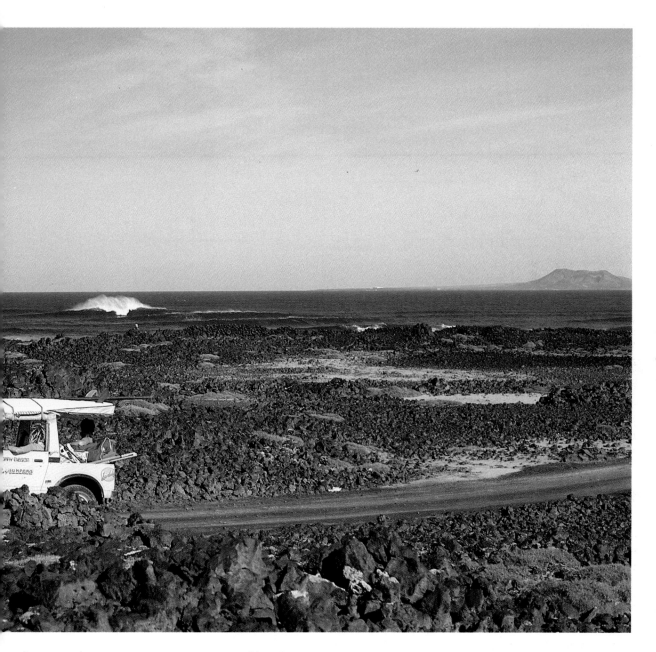

Lanzarote

Lanzarote is the neighbouring island to Fuerteventura, and has the same black volcanic appearance. Its capital is Puerto del Carmen, which is a big holiday centre, and the two nearby beaches of Los Poscillos and Matagorda both offer good, moderate short board conditions.

Other launch spots are few and far between. Las Salinas offers a reef break near its rocky harbour entrance and for true hotshots the north-facing Famara Bay is a magnificent location pounded by huge dumping waves.

Gran Canaria

The two main spots are the resort complex of Bahia Feliz where Club Mistral have a holiday and board hire operation for their whole range. A few miles up the coast Pozo guarantees strong winds and good waves, but launching over the municipal rubbish dump is not particularly lovely.

Tenerife

Tenerife's main windsurfing location is El Medano on the south-east corner of the island. It's a small village just five miles from the airport, and is rated as one of the best spots in the Canaries.

Columbia Gorge

Each spring the Columbia Gorge Pro-Am Slalom takes place at Hood River, attracting the world's best short board competition sailors and rating as one of their top 10 events in the international calendar.

The Columbia River stretches from British Columbia, through the border, and snakes down through Washington State to empty into the Pacific Ocean on the Oregon coast. However, it is the part of the river known as the 'Gorge' which is important to windsurfers, because the coastal winds funnel directly up its length.

When Portland City is cloudy and cool and the Gorge has clear skies, the pressure difference created draws air through a gap in the Cascade Mountains creating a squeeze effect on the wind. The wind then blows at between 15–40 knots along the Gorge, and while the river flows from east to west, the wind blows from west to east and pushes up an amazing swell which can be jumped on both port and starboard tacks.

Seasonal Conditions
The season starts around the beginning of March, and tapers off during September when it becomes too cold to sail. The best times to visit are the summer months from May to August, when there is usually at least 20 days per month with the right kind of high winds for excellent short board sailing.

The water is likely to be a cool 38–45°F in spring, caused by the snow melting in the mountains, with strong currents.

Towards July you can expect the water temperatures to rise to around 70°F with air temperatures in the 80–90°F range, but even so most Gorge sailors wear a wetsuit all year round.

You have to be willing to drive around to find the right place with sailing conditions that suit your sailing abilities. It might be blowing hard in one spot while it's only five knots just a few miles down the river.

The winds are unpredictable, and in fact the United Telephone Company have a recorded message *Wind Line* which gives daily readings for the various areas as well as a general forecast which is updated every hour.

Other Attractions
If you miss the wind, you can drive up through the Mount Hood National Forest Park which is incredibly beautiful, and then head up to the 11,260 foot high Mount Hood which is some 40 miles to the south, and is the focal point of the Gorge.

Mount Hood has the only year-round skiing in the USA, and ski hire equipment and lift passes up to the 8,000 foot high runs are readily available. Where else can you go skiing in the morning and wave-sailing in the afternoon?

If that doesn't suit you the area

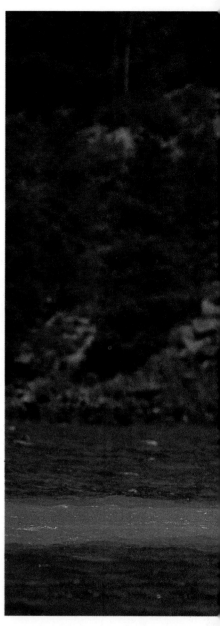

Above: Action on the Gorge during a Pro-Am Slalom, the annual event which attracts the world's top sailors.

Left: There is a wide choice of sailing spots along the Gorge from which to select a suitable launch site. For high winds the best locations are Hood River Marina, Swell City, Home Valley Park, Doug's Beach, Avery Park, and Maryhill State Park on the Washington side.

COLUMBIA RIVER GORGE
WASHINGTON

Home Valley Swell City Bingen Maryhill
Doug's Beach Avery Park
Hood River

OREGON

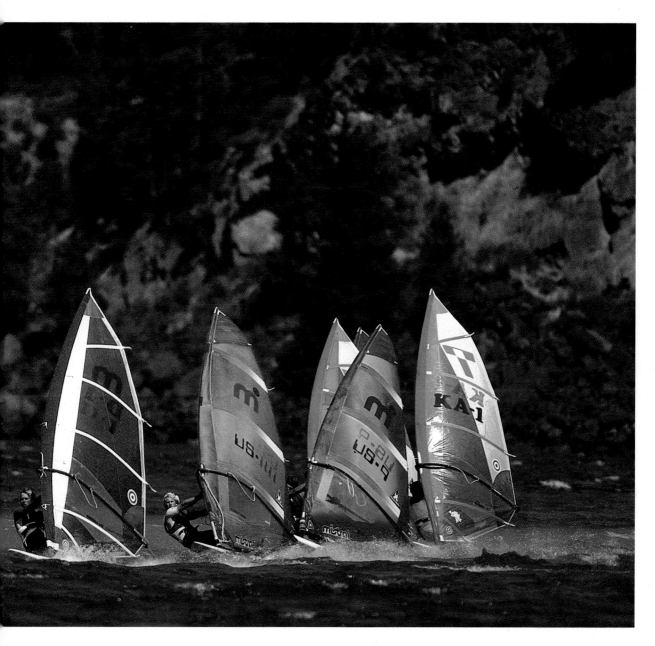

is excellent for trekking, fishing, white water rafting, kayaking, or mountain biking. You need never be at a loss if the wind fails.

Sailing in the Gorge

With the wind going one way and the current the other, you never have to sail upwind to get back to your departure point. The width of the river varies from a quarter of a mile to a mile, and the uninter-rupted broad reaches from side to side are very fast and exciting, with the possibility of swells up to head high in the centre.

The technique for jumping in the Gorge is best described as an upwind jump, which means that you have to crank the board into the wind before you get airborne off a wave. The backdrop to the sailing is beautiful, and being on a broad reach all the time means that you have no worries about getting your board upwind.

With all its other facilities the Columbia Gorge is truly a wind-surfers' paradise. The only things to look out for are the barges which run up and down the river; the gill nets which are laid close to the shore; and the fines if the police catch you without a 'personal flotation device' which is required by law.

The West Country

The UK undoubtedly has the best short board sailing in northern Europe. It also has some very good waves, whereas the Mediterranean has none that could be described as 'big'. On the debit side, alas, the weather can be very cold and the wind is unpredictable.

The most dependable times of year are spring and autumn, with the latter being marginally more favourable since the sea has had time to heat up to something better than freezing! Obviously steamer style wetsuits are mandatory for any kind of short board sailing.

The Atlantic Influence

The best areas all face west, where short board sailors benefit from the long uninterrupted fetch which builds up the waves that accompany the winds from mid Atlantic.

In the far north, the Scottish island of Tiree is famed as the windiest place in Britain and has some excellent wavesailing spots. Unfortunately it is also remote and inaccessible.

Further south much of the Welsh coastline has excellent wind and wave conditions, with many ideal sideshore locations. Amongst the best known are the Isle of Anglesey where principal spots are Rhosneigr and Trearddur Bay; and Dyfedd in the south where Newgale, Broadhaven, Pendine and Amroth are all recommended for short boards.

However, it is 'The Wild West' that is Britain's capital of short board sailing.

'The Wild West'

This is Devon and Cornwall, the adjoining counties which receive the best of the strong south-westerlies and have some formidable swells. Before windsurfing took off this area was famous for surfing. Now the two sports co-exist and have spawned a score or more of well known custom and short board manufacturing firms, as well as excellent sailmakers and wetsuit and accessory manufacturers.

Established names include New Waves, Circle One and Chapter – all making short boards in Devon; Vitamin Sea, Light Waves and Limited Edition provide the same service over the border in Cornwall.

You will also find Gul, Hy Jumpers, Cosmic, Tornado, Second Skin, Tiki, Lodey and many others who are dedicated to serving the needs of the short board sailor.

Best Spots

On the south Devon coastline, Bantham and Bigbury which face one another across a single bay are best known for advanced wavesailing; but, on those out of control days, Mothercombe and Salcombe offer more protected conditions. Wembury is good if the prevailing south-westerly swings round to the north-west, and all of these

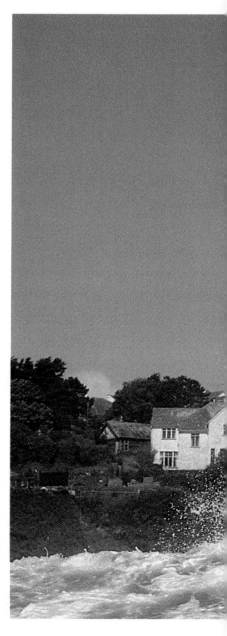

Above: Local sailor Duncan Lawson shows what it's like off the south Devon coastline. Photographer Alex Williams has the advantage of living close to the cliffs of Bigbury Bay, where this picture was taken.

Left: The Wild West. The Devon/Cornwall peninsula is ideally angled and positioned to make the most of the prevailing south-westerly winds. The short board spots are shown.

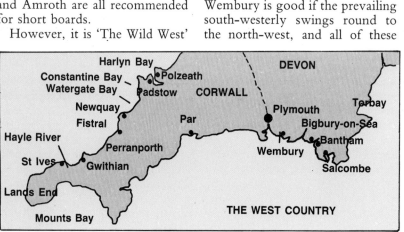

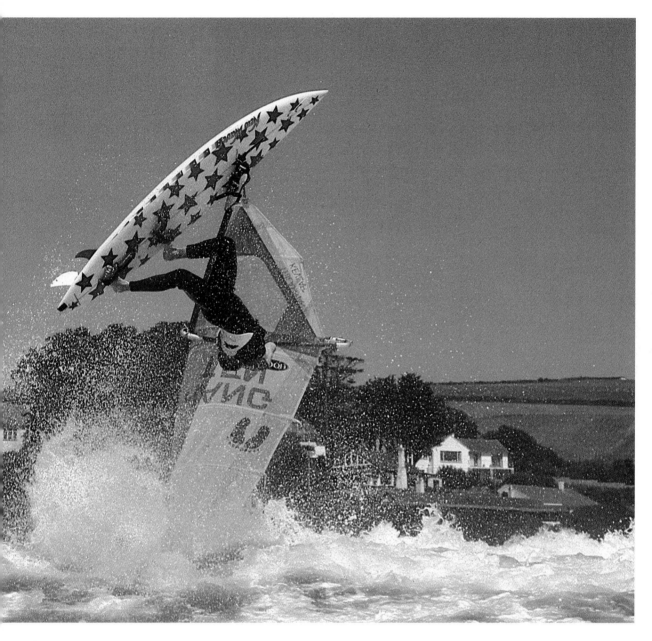

places are pretty areas to sail in, quiet and uncrowded – *outside* the peak summer holiday times.

Over the border, the wave spots on the south Cornish coast are few and far between, with Par and the spectacular Mounts Bay (it has a castle in the middle) best known.

However, it's only 20 miles at most to the north coast, so if the south fails a short drive through attractive country will give you the choice of the Hayle rivermouth, Perranporth, Watergate, Fistral, Constantine, Harlyn or Polzeath. All are highly rated for advanced sailing.

Cross the border into north Devon, and it's a couple of hours' drive along the slow, winding roads before you reach the Braunton and Saunton area which is notable for its concentration of windsurfing related manufacturers and small businesses.

The beaches of Saunton and neighbouring Croyde are patronised by both surfers and short board sailors. If there isn't any wind, there are large expanses of hard packed sand at low tide; ideal for practising short board manoeuvres with a Speed Sail (see page 120).

The South West Funboard Cup (autumn) is the area's main event.

Glossary of Short Board Terms

Board, Rig and Sailor

A
Asymmetric
Boards with asymmetric tail shapes first appeared in 1983, and are primarily used in Hawaii and in particular at Hookipa where the break is always the same. A great exponent of the asymmetric is Craig Masonville who produces Hi Tech custom boards on Oahu. The basic idea is that the bottom turn side is long and drawn out for high speed turns at the bottom of the wave; while the cut back side is wide and floaty for slower turns off the top of the wave.

B
Battens
Tapered full length battens are necessary to maintain a draught forward shape in a rotational sail. The best are hand laminated and are expensive. Machine made extruded battens tend to have less effective taper, but maintain adequate stability when used with camber inducers.

Bevel
A bevelled rail is cut off at an angle to compromise between a hard and soft rail shape. The bevel is sometimes concave to give a quattro concave effect for marginal planing.

Blind Stitch
The blind stitch stitches the neoprene panels of a wetsuit together without piercing them. Most steamers are stitched in this way for minimum water penetration.

Boom
Fixed length booms tend to be stiffest, but most sailors prefer to compromise with a good quality adjustable boom which covers a wide range of sail sizes. Telescopic extensions are generally more adaptable and convenient than removable extension pieces.

A soft rubber boom grip is generally favoured (Pro Grip etc), but this wears badly and may need replacing after a couple of seasons – a long and quite difficult job which is best left to the specialist or DIY enthusiast.

The boom angle at the inhaul end must be suitable for your sail. At least 65° is usually necessary to accommodate the camber in contemporary sails.

C
Camber Inducer
A plastic moulding, shaped like a tuning fork, which attaches the full length batten directly to the mast. It induces perfect camber and excellent rotational characteristics. Very good for power and speed, very poor for manoeuvrability due to the ultra stable shape of the sail.

Carbon
Carbon is used in skin laminates for both custom and moulded board production. It has excellent stiffness, strength and torsional properties; but it is difficult to work with and prohibitively expensive. It tends to appear only as carbon strip or carbon/glass reinforcement.

Concaves
It is generally accepted that concaves make boards go faster, accelerating the air from nose to tail as the board rides on it like a cushion.

Most speed orientated short boards have a single concave (sometimes double) nose for lift to promote initial planing; and a double concave midsection tapering into very slight concaves or flats at the tail. The depth of the concaves is critical, with deeper concaves generally better in stronger winds when their pronounced V helps break up chop.

There are many concave variations – treble, quattro, and multi channel boards.

Custom
A custom board is a one-off, hand rather than machine made. However, some custom boards are more one-off than others, with the great majority being made from templates to more or less identical shapes. Once tried, most short board sailors find that a custom feels better than a moulded board, possibly helped by the fact that it inevitably looks more attractive.

Custom sails, custom fins, etc are also produced along the same individual lines.

D
Downhaul
The amount of downhaul required will generally depend on the type of sail and the stiffness of the mast. On most rotationals and camber induced sails a hard pull with 3:1 purchase is all that is necessary. Too much downhaul will prevent a sail from rotating.

E
Epoxy
Epoxy is widely used to produce light, stiff skin laminates made up of composite materials or glassfibre.

In custom construction it is less popular as it is difficult to laminate. So polyester resin laminates with polyurethane foam tend to be the favourite material.

Epoxy can be used with polyurethane or polystyrene; polyester can be used with polyurethane but not with polystyrene which it will melt.

F
Flats
Flat areas on the bottom of the board.

Fins
Fins stop the board going sideways. Narrow tail boards which have good grip on the water require less fin area than wide tail boards, which is why the latter tend to have three fins.

Designers are always searching for the ultimate fin which won't spin out due to losing its grip on the water.

Fin Boxes
Fin boxes are machine made in uniform sizes of different lengths. All fins should be interchangeable, but depending on the construction of the board, some mouldings squeeze the box or boxes and others make a very loose fit. Fin boxes are also used as mast tracks for most custom boards.

Footstraps
Should be adjustable (usually with Velcro), comfortable (with thick neoprene outer padding), and correctly placed for optimum trim and control of the board. Some boards feature an asymmetric strap arrangement for jumping and riding.

G/H

Handles
Should be found at the clew which helps with outhaul tension; and at the head of the sail for holding on in wipe-outs.

Harness
The inventor deserves a Nobel Prize for coming up with the windsurfer's best friend. Seat and waist harnesses tend to be favoured for short board speed sailing with a low hook sitting-down position; while a higher hook gives more security for difficult wavesailing.

I

Inhaul
Must be rigid, but take great care not to crush the mast when rigging – guarantee claims won't cover it.

J/K/L

Leash
Leashing the rig to the board gets widely overlooked, but is every bit as important as a surfer leashing the board to his foot. There comes a time when the board and rig are parted, and you may be unable to catch the board on its own.

Leech
The trailing edge of the sail from the head to the clew. The leech must always be supported by battens.

Luff
The leading edge of the sail from the head to the tack where it meets the mastfoot. The luff tube attaches the sail to the mast.

M

Mastfoot
The mastfoot unit is attached to the board via the powerjoint. Many use a simple mast plate which is bolted to a fin box in the deck. One or two bolts hold it in position, and it is simply adjusted on the beach.

Mast Protector
A neoprene buffer which is fastened round the foot of the mast in order to protect the deck. Well worth using, particularly on more fragile custom boards.

Mast Track
Many moulded short boards have an adjustable mast track, which is useful for making quick and easy adjustments out on the water. The shorter the board the less it becomes necessary and the greater the weight penalty.

N/O

Outhaul
Fully battened sails tend to need very little outhaul tension, particularly camber induced sails which will lose all their power if over outhauled.

P

Polyester
Polyester resin is much used to make custom boards with PU foam cores. It cannot be used with polystyrene foam. The rival merits and demerits of polyester and epoxy resin tend to be hotly debated, but neither is clearly superior.

Polystyrene (EPS)
EPS foam is light and brittle when compared to PU. It is much used to make high volume boards. With low volume custom boards weight is not so critical and more durable PU is usually preferred.

Polyurethane (PU)
PU foam is heavier and more durable than EPS. Most custom blanks are made in PU, with leading brand names such as Clark from the USA and Phenolic Megalite from Australia.

Q/R

Rails
Rails vary from soft to hard along the sides of the board. They are called rails because the board runs on them, and if they're straight it will go straight. That's why you gybe on the curve of the tail.

Rotational
Barry Spanier and Jeff Bourne invented the rotational in 1984. There are countless rotational sails on the market, but some rotate more than others. The problem is that all rotationals will start to de-rotate in a very strong wind, which has the effect of shifting an area of unwanted cloth back in the sail. Generally the more battens a rotational sail has, the more stable it will be.

A good rotational is the best sail for most short board uses, from flat water speed to moderate wave control.

S

Slalom
Short board racing round a series of closely spaced marks.

Soft Sails
Sails are soft when their main body is unsupported by full length battens. They tend to have two or three short battens in the leech to maintain the roach, and a full length batten in the head and foot.

Apart from being light, the main advantage of a soft sail is that you can turn off the power instantly when riding on a big wave face.

Speed Trials
The fastest board timed over a 500 metre course. There are half a dozen major international speed events each year.

Steamer
The steamer is the right wetsuit for 99 per cent of short board sailors who sail in cold waters. The seams are dry (usually with blind stitching), and with a tight fit at neck, ankles and wrists, very little water can get in so that the occupant keeps really warm. A drysuit will be warmer, but tends to be bulky for short board use.

Stringers
Longitudinals, usually made of plywood, which are used to give the board stiffness and strength throughout its length. Virtually all custom boards are stringered; while because of problems with construction most moulded boards are not. A custom board may be fragile on the outside, but it's very strong on the inside!

T

Tinkler Tail
A 1985 development seen on some custom boards. The tail is spring-loaded, and the amount of flex can be adjusted to compensate for sailing in a chop. The idea came from surfing, but is as yet unproven in windsurfing.

Thrusters
The small fins on either side of the main fin.

Tuck
A rail is tucked when it is cut away on an angle to compromise between hard and soft.

U/V

V Bottom
V in the bottom gives grip against loss of lateral resistance. Most short boards have a small amount of V in the tail, as well as V created by double concaves in the mid section.

Velcro
Where would we be without it? Much used for adjustable footstraps, mast protectors, and other short board hardware.

Volume
The overall amount of volume helps determine whether the board will be a floater, marginal or sinker. Volume distribution has a marked effect on the board's performance.

W

Wave Performance
A wave competition, divided between riding in with the waves, jumping out through them, and transitions on the inside and outside.

Wide Point
The wide point of a board helps determine its outline, and has a marked effect on its tail shape.

Glossary of Short Board Terms

Sailing Terms

A

Aerial
Any manoeuvre performed up in the air.

Apparent Wind
The wind direction and speed created by the board's forward motion.

B

Backside
Riding with your back to the wave.

Bale Out
Leave the board in mid air.

Beach Start
Carry your board and rig into the water, hop on, and sail off.

Beating
Sailing as close to the wind as possible.

Body Drag
Hopping off the board to drag your body in the water for a few seconds.

Bottom Turn
Bearing away at the bottom of the wave to ride up again.

Bowling
The top of the wave starts to bowl over and form a tube.

Break
Where the waves pitch up and break due to the lessening depth of water.

C

Carve
Carving a turn is banking the board like a ski, and letting it turn on the curve of the tail.

Chop
Small waves created by the wind.

Clew-first
Riding with the rig reversed, clew-first to the wind. It usually happens when coming out a gybe.

Close Out
The wave breaks along its entire length, usually in an offshore wind.

Cross-shore
The wind blowing from left to right or right to left is best for windsurfing, giving a beam reach out and back again.

Cut-back
You cut back at the top of the wave to head back down the face again.

D

Depression
Usually indicates a period of unsettled weather, and in colder climates frequently means wind.

Donkey Kick
Kicking the board out sideways in mid-air.

Drop-in
Getting the board on to a wave face.

Duck Gybe
Gybing under the boom.

Dumper
A wave that breaks fiercely on a steeply shelving shoreline, often with a dangerous undertow.

E

Eye of the wind
The direction the wind is coming from.

F

Footsteer
Using your feet to weight the inner or outer rail to steer the board.

Freestyle
There are a number of short board freestyle tricks, including tail-first tacks, helicopters, duck gybes etc.

Frontside
Riding with your front to the wave.

G

Gnarly
Waves that are peaking and breaking all over the place.

Groundswell
Waves created by ocean depressions. They travel many hundreds of miles before peaking and breaking when they reach shallow water.

Gybing
Altering course so the tail of the board passes through the eye of the wind.

H

Head Up
To steer the board up into the wind.

Helicopter
Freestyle trick involving pushing the rig round through 180 degrees to tack.

Hypothermia
Dangerous condition of extreme cold brought on by wind chill and water temperature.

J

Jumping
If the wave is steep enough and you're fast enough, the board just has to jump.

K

Knots
Nautical miles per hour – the way in which speed is recorded on water. A nautical mile measures 2000 yards (1.65 km).

L

Late Drop
Leaving it until the last moment to drop down the face of the wave as it's breaking.

Leeward
Sideways drift due to lack of lateral resistance of the fin or board.

I

Inside
Inside the break, when sailing close to the beach.

Left Break
The wave breaks to the left of the surfer or sailor.

Le Mans Start
A slalom start from the beach.

Lip
The top of the wave where it is starting to break.

Loop
Jumping the board and looping it right round for a perfect landing. If the loop is more horizontal, it is called a *barrel roll*.

Low
Another word for depression.

Luffing
Heading up into the wind; or letting the sail out to depower it.

M

Man-on-man
Two competitors sailing against one another, usually in a wave performance competition.

Munched
Falling and being pummelled by a wave.

Mush
Small, breaking waves with a lot of white water.

N/O

Offshore Wind
Blowing away from the shore; this wind is usually good for surfing since it holds up the waves.

Off the Lip
Turning off the breaking lip of the wave. An aerial off the lip is performed in mid-air.

Onshore
A wind blowing on to the shore, which makes it difficult to sail away from the launch place.

Outside
Outside the break, when sailing far away from the beach.

Over the Falls
Being thrown out by the lip of the wave.

P

Peeling
A wave peels when it breaks gradually along its length.

Plane
The board skims on top of the water, cutting down its wetted surface area for maximum speed.

Port
Port hand is left, denoted by the colour red. Except in some waveriding applications, port tack (when windward is the port side) always gives way to starboard tack.

Pump
Vigorously rocking the rig back and forth to create more apparent wind to get the board moving.

Q/R

Reach
Sail with the wind on the beam.

Reef Break
When the waves pile up and break on a reef.

Rip
The water coming in with the waves is carried out by the rip. This can be dangerous if the rip moves very fast.

Run
Sailing with the wind behind. There is no pull from the leeward side of the sail, and it is not an efficient direction on a short board.

S

Set
Waves travel as a set, like a platoon of soldiers.

Shorebreak
When waves break on the shore, due to the lessening depth of water.

Shoulder
The part of the wave which has not broken.

Sideshore
The same as *Cross-shore*.

Spin-out
When the fin ventilates or cavitates, it loses its grip on the water and the tail slides away from under the sailor.

Starboard
The right hand side, denoted by the colour green. Starboard tack (when the windward side is the right side) has right of way over port tack.

Surfing
Using the steepness of a wave face to gather momentum and ride it.

T

Tack
Turning the board so the nose passes through the eye of the wind. Seldom used on short boards, due to lack of flotation and space in the nose.

Three-sixty
Carving the board round through a full 360 degrees on the water.

Tide
Coastal movements of water induced by the pull of sun and moon.

Top Turn
As for *Cut back* – turning off the top of the wave.

Transition
A change in direction from tack to tack – usually a gybe.

Traverse
Sailing along a wave face.

Trim
Both sail and board are trimmed for maximum effect, using feet, hands and body weight.

True Wind
The true direction the wind is coming from.

Tube
When the lip of the wave pitches right over it leaves a hollow tube in the middle. Top surfers can ride along this tube.

U

Upside Down
Kicking the board upside down in a jump – also called a table top.

V

Ventilation
Similar to *Cavitation*. Air gets round the fin, so it loses its grip on the water.

W

Waterstart
Using the rig to pull the sailor up out of the water and on to the board.

Wave Ride
Catching a wave, and riding on its face.

Wetted Area
The wetted surface area of the bottom of the board is proportional to the amount of drag. The less the wetted area the faster the board will go, which is why small boards are fastest.

Windshift
A change in the wind's direction. There are small windshifts every moment when you are sailing.

Windward
The side the wind is blowing towards. The windward rail is also called the *outer rail*.

Wipe-out
Fall off and wipe-out before starting all over again!

Appendix I
Weather

The Beaufort Scale
The wind is measured on the Beaufort Scale, invented by Admiral Sir Francis Beaufort in 1805. The units are knots, which are nautical miles (about 1.85 kilometres) per hour. These descriptions are for life on the open sea. It won't be quite so extreme close inshore, which is windsurfer territory.

Force 0
1 knot or less. Calm. Mirror-like sea.

Force 1
1–3 knots. Light air. Gently scaly ripples.

Force 2
4–6 knots. Light breeze. Small wavelets. May have glassy crests but these will not break.

Force 3
7–10 knots. Gentle breeze: large wavelets. Crests begin to break. Possibly some white horses.

Force 4
11–16 knots. Moderate breeze. Waves becoming longer with white horses.

Force 5
17–21 knots. Fresh breeze. Moderate waves with white horses and possibly occasional spray.

Force 6
22–27 knots. Strong breeze. Large waves forming with extensive white crests and spray.

Force 7
28–33 knots. Near gale. Sea heaps up and foam from breaking waves blows in streaks.

Force 8
34–40 knots. Gale. Moderately high waves. Edge of crests break into spindrift. Well marked streaks.

Force 9
41–47 knots. Severe gale. High waves. Confused breaking crests. Spray affects visibility.

Force 10
48–55 knots. Storm. Very high waves with long overhanging crests. Sea surface becomes white.

Force 11
56–63 knots. Violent storm Exceptionally high waves hiding ships from view. Sea covered in white foam.

Force 12
64 knots plus. Hurricane. Air full of driving spray. Very bad visibility.

Weather Forecasts
Weather forecasts are available on the TV, radio and in the newspapers. The TV and newspaper forecasts usually show expected wind speeds and directions, but are for people on land.

The most useful forecasts are often found on the radio. Local coastal radio stations generally have accurate news of wind and sea state which is useful if you live in the area; otherwise you will have to make do with national radio which best serves windsurfers with the forecast for inshore waters broadcast on Radio 3 weekday mornings at 0655 (early enough to get you down to the coast in good time), and weekends at 0755. For late birds an alternative time for the inshore forecast is 0038 on Radio 4 LW.

As an alternative you can try the *Shipping Forecast* broadcast on Radio 4 LW at 0033, 0555, 1355 and 1750. It gives a good general picture, but the information relates more to the open sea where conditions may be very different from those experienced by a windsurfer close inshore.

If you're not organised enough to catch any of the above, there are a variety of telephone forecasts. In the back of your Telephone Dialing Codes booklet you will find the numbers of recorded message forecasts, but a better alternative is probably the RYA's *Marineline* designed specifically for yachtsmen:
1. **Channel**: Brighton 0273 550266; Portsmouth 0705 861144; Southampton 0703 336161; Bournemouth 0202 295588.
2. **South-West**: Plymouth 0792 8092; Truro 0872 41717.
3. **Bristol Channel**: Bristol 0272 291050; Swansea 0792 42020; Weston Super Mare 0934 419468.
4. **Wales**: Aberystwyth 0970 611822; Bangor 0248 354900.
5. **North-West**: Liverpool 051–236 2060; Douglas IOM 0624 77070.
6. **Ulster**: Belfast 0232 234400.
7. **Clyde**: Ayr 0292 286000; Glasgow 041–552 4466.
8. **Caledonia**: Glasgow 041–552 4477; Oban 0631 66000.
9. **Minch**: Ullapool 0854 2757.
10. **Pentland**: Thurso 0595 4640.
11. **Scotland East**: Inverness 0463 234260; Edinburgh 031–225 3232; Dundee 0382 737741.
12. **East**: Newcastle-upon-Tyne 0632 324466; Cleethorpes 0472 603603; Scarborough 0723 35377.
13. **East Anglia**: Great Yarmouth 0493 855655; Southend 0702 333444; Medway 0634 44544; London 01–671 6363.

Rather than listen to a recording, you may want specific advice. You can try phoning the *Coastguard* (look in the Directory) who can advise on prevailing conditions. Alternatively the men who run *Weather Centres* can tell you what sort of windsurfing weather to expect. Queuing systems apply and you sometimes have to wait a long time before your call is answered:

London Weather Centre
01–836 4311
Southampton Weather Centre
0703 28844
Plymouth Meteorological Centre
0752 82534
Cardiff Airport
0446 710343
Manchester Weather Centre
061–832 6701
Glasgow Weather Centre
041–248 3451
Lerwick Meteorological Office
0595 2293

Appendix II
Travel

Flying with a Board
If you decide to take your own board and equipment to some foreign shore, do your homework.

Most aircraft have holds which are big enough to take boards, but that does not mean to say they will. The travel agent may assure you that you can just turn up at the check-in and everything will be OK, but unless he is a windsurfing specialist it is best to contact the airline, and if possible get their agreement in writing. Most will agree to take boards and many will do so free of charge.

Full length masts are frequently a problem, and it is much easier to travel with a two-part mast – there are some excellent ones on the market.

How to Arrange the Trip
1. Check that your insurance is valid for the country in question.
2. Wrap the board. It's usually best to tape (use wide brown tape) the boom and sails to the deck, which helps protect it and leaves you less to carry. The rails should be heavily protected (try cardboard) after which the whole board should be covered in bubble wrap – two layers – and securely taped. Remember to carry enough tape for the homeward journey.

If you travel frequently, it will be worth investing in a proper board bag. The best are expensive, but they are tough enough to protect your board on a plane trip.
3. Arrive at the airport early, ready to be the first to check-in. Grab two trolleys, lay the board across them, and you will be able to push it on your own. Tell the check-in staff that you have a board, they should send baggage handlers to fetch it.
4. On arrival at your destination there may be Customs problems. Some countries demand a deposit on the value of your gear which is refundable when you leave. You should be able to find out in advance how much they are likely to require.
5. If you need a roof rack and straps, don't forget to take them. You can't stick a board in the back seat of a taxi!

Appendix III

Build Your Own Custom Board

DIY 2.50 metre Gun

To build this board you need to assemble:

Tools

Steel tape measure
Set square
Spirit level
Paint roller and tray
Stanley knife
Jigsaw
Spokeshave
Electric drill
Power plane
Scissors
Bench vice
'Hot wire'

Materials

1 suitably sized block of Styrofoam (stronger and marginally more easy to work with than similar polystyrene, but more expensive). For the board shown the size should be 260 cm × 600 cm × 150 cm.
1 sheet plywood, 4 mm thick × 2.50 m long, to make a central stringer to be bonded in place down the middle of the foam.
4 litres epoxy resin/hardener
13 metres Woven glass cloth 200 gsm
5.2 metres carbon fibre, 30 cm wide
2 skeg boxes for fin and mast track
2 mixing pots and sticks
2 pairs disposable gloves
Particle mask
2 in brush
Squeegee
Roll of masking tape

Design

If you are making your own design, draw plan, profile and lateral cross section on graph paper using a scale of 1mm square to 1cm of board.

Templates

Plot 10cm squares on an 8ft × 4ft sheet of hardboard using a tape, straight edge, and pencil. Number them for clarity, and then plot a full size half plan from the drawing on the graph paper. To do this use a biro and ruler to plot each point where the shape passes through the boxes of the graph paper. These points are then trans-ferred to the corresponding positions on the hardboard. When you have finished use a thick felt pen and the outside of a bent flexible edge (try a plastic curtain rail or batten) to draw the curve which joins all the points. Two people are needed to do this, and it helps if nails are used to hold the flexible edge in position.

Do the same with the profile, always taking bottom and deck measurements from the same longitudinal line.

The next stage is to cut out both templates, which takes time and patience. A useful tip is to use the edge of the hardboard as the straight centre line of the half plan – you will never be able to cut such a straight line yourself. Use a jigsaw, and take utmost care to stay on the outside of the lines.

Halving the foam block

To make a 'hot wire' all that is required is a 2in × 2in wooden framework with old electric heater filament wire strung tightly across and wound around a couple of nails on each side of the frame. Run a pair of jump leads from the nails to a car battery or battery charger, and you have a safe and effective cutting machine. Take your foam block and turn it on edge. Resting your hot wire on the top of the foam and keeping it square, slice a straight line along the length of the block, thus cutting it in half. Having two people to hold the hot wire makes a more accurate job.

Cutting the profile

Take one of the halves of the foam block, and draw round the template profile on the two sides of the block. Next take your hot wire and cut around the profile outline. Repeat exactly the same process with the other half of the foam block.

Stringering

Draw the outline of your profile template onto the ply provided for the stringer. Cut out the ply and fair the edges until it is oversized all round by 1–2mm.

Mix approximately 150cc of resin and hardener (follow the manufacturer's instructions – a syringe is useful for measuring small quantities), and stir thoroughly. Use a 2 inch brush to coat all the surfaces to be joined, and then place the stringer between the halves of the block making sure there is nowhere that the stringer is proud of the foam – the blocks and stringer will remain easy to adjust for about 30 minutes, so take your time. When you are satisfied clamp the stringer between the foam using roof rack straps. The blank must now be left for at least eight hours.

Cutting the plan outline

Lay the half plan template on the stringered top of the blank with the straight edge along the stringer. Draw a line around the outside, and turn the template over and repeat the process on the opposite side. If the straight edge of the template remains aligned along the stringer, this will give you a perfect symmetrical shape. Unfortunately the rocker which has been cut into the blank will not allow the template to lie perfectly flat, which makes marking the outline a little more difficult.

Now cut away the surplus foam with the hot wire, taking care to cut square or obliquely away from the centre of the blank, and always outside the outline.

Shaping

1. Take the bottom side down to the stringer. Work at first with an electric plane or surform, and then with a long sanding block. (A 3ft long flat wooden block with fine grade 100 sandpaper stapled or glued on one side and rough grade 40 on the other is the ideal tool.) Check continually with a spirit level and by eye to ensure that the surface is flat and even. If you need to cut the stringer down, use a very small plane or spokeshave.

2. Turn the blank over and repeat this process on the deck.

3. Re-mark the outline of the half plan template on the blank. Turn the blank on edge, and surform and sand the top edge down to within 1–2mm of its eventual size, while using a set square to maintain a 90 degree angle between the deck/bottom and sides. Leave the ends (nose and tail) until last. Treat them carefully as they are fragile and difficult to shape symmetrically.

4. Turn the blank over and repeat the process on the other side.

5. Typically you will be looking to shape a shallow V in the tail which will have hard, sharp edges leading into a more rounded rail profile further forward. Without going into details you should draw accurate measured lines which correspond to your rail shapes along the edges and top and bottom of the blank, and then surform down to them until you have a succession of flat, narrow planes forming the curve of rails and deck. You can then work with a long sheet of sandpaper (one end in each hand) to give a rounded curve to the rails. Work on the rails from the bottom first before turning the board to work from the deck.

6. On the bottom of the blank draw an oblong representing the furthest extent of a single area of concave (if desired). Reduce the stringer with a spokeshave, and then working outwards take down the foam with a small, slightly rounded sanding block.

7. You can use the same methods to form double concaves.

8. Finish the blank by sanding all over with fine grade 180 sandpaper.

Laminating the bottom

Make sure the room you are working in is as dust free as possible, and that the temperature is above 18°C. Lay the cloth (200gsm woven rovings) along the bottom of the board and cut it with a 5cm length overlap. Then use scissors to cut around the shape of the board, leaving a similar overlap. Carefully roll up the cloth from one end, and put it aside. Repeat this with a second layer of cloth.

Take some good quality non-absorbent masking tape and fix it around the edge of the board approximately 3cm beyond the rails of the side you intend to laminate – this is necessary to allow for an overlap of cloth on a very vulnerable area. Fix second and third strips of tape further round – they are there to prevent resin dripping onto the side you're not laminating.

Put on gloves and/or barrier cream. Prepare the resin and hardener according to the manufacturer's instructions (about 1 litre per side) and mix very thoroughly, adding colour pigment if required. Apply a thin coat of resin to the foam.

Unroll the first layer of glass cloth onto the foam, and smooth it out with your hands, adjusting its overall position. Roll more resin into the glass until it is completely 'wetted out'.

Then, using a squeegee and working from slightly beyond the centreline, scrape the resin towards the sides, taking care not to lift or drag the glass.

When you have worked all the air and excess resin out of the glass, wet out the rails using a roller or paint brush and then squeegee them. Immediately you finish, unroll the second layer of glass on top of the first and repeat the process.

Where the rails are very sharp, the glass will not want to stay stuck down. The solution is to tape it down with masking tape which is fixed across the other side of the board.

The *Aerotex* carbon fibre strip is laminated in at the same time and in the same way, and can be put above, beneath, or between the layers of glassfibre. Squeegee out along the grain of the longitudinal carbon strands for the best effect. Finally, wash all the tools with acetone. Unless you do this immediately, they will become useless.

'Cutting off'

Two or three hours after laminating, while the fibreglass is still a bit tacky take a Stanley knife with a sharp blade and cut through the glass along the inner layer of masking tape. Peel off the tape and redundant laminate.

Laminating the deck

Allow the bottom to cure for at least eight hours before turning it over to repeat the process on the deck. The deck usually requires a third layer of glass to reinforce it against the foot loads it has to bear. You can add small extra layers of cloth to any particularly vulnerable areas – nose, mastfoot, footstraps, etc.

Artwork

Wait eight hours after the final lamination. Sand the surface with wet & dry (down to 180 grade) to give yourself a smoothish surface to work on, and then clean it with acetone and wipe dry. The colours you apply will later be sealed and protected by the gel coat and varnish.

Footstraps

Neoprene covered Velcro adjustable straps can either be glassed or screwed into the deck. In common with the skeg and mast foot boxes this process

can be carried out before or after applying the flow coat.

Mark the chosen position for the straps, and cut out very thin slits to a depth of about 4cm with a jigsaw, making sure that the ends of the straps can be slid in and out but are still a tight fit. The slits for each strap should be about 15cm apart. Having cut the slits, mask up to the edges with tape and paper, and then mix your resin. For any fittings it is advisable to use an additive known as 'glass bubbles' which thickens the resin for an easier and better job.

Half fill the slits with the mixed resin and poke in the straps. Wipe away excess resin that is pushed out and leave to harden before removing the masking tape. Do not attempt to make up the strap for at least eight hours.

If you're using screw fixings, glass in two purpose made Rawlplugs for each strap end, using a drill to make the holes. When the resin has hardened, fix the strap with two stainless steel screws which should pass through a plastic plate in order to spread the load and prevent the webbing tearing.

Mastfoot fin boxes

Mark the exact position of the necessary slot or slots, according to the fin box system you intend to use. Cut out the glassfibre with a jigsaw and the foam with a router or Stanley knife and file. Check that the slot you make is exactly the size of the fin box.

Mask around the slot and over the top of the box. Use the same resin mix as for the straps, quarter fill the slot, and insert the box so that it is exactly flush with the deck. Wipe off excess resin and allow time for curing.

Flow coat

The flow coat is basically a further coat of resin (also called a 'gel coat') which seals the board and the artwork. The application is similar to a top coat of gloss paintwork. Leave the flow coat for eight hours to cure, before turning the board over and starting on the bottom.

Varnishing

You may wish to give the board a coat of *SP 2000* two-part polyurethane varnish over the flow coat. It will counteract the effect of UV light and will protect the colours in your board for that much longer, and it is non porous.

Non-slip

Mask off the non-slip area, bearing in mind where you will be standing. Sand and rub the surface with acetone. Apply a coat of resin and hardener (colloidal silica is not required for this process). While the resin is still wet, and without waiting for it to go tacky, sprinkle liberal quantities of salt or sugar evenly over the whole area.

Sanding & polishing

Use wet and dry sandpaper, rubbing evenly and lightly. You might start with 180 grade, and finish using a very fine 400 or 600 grade paper – the more you rub and the finer the grade, the better the finish will be.

After sanding the polishing can begin. First apply 'rubbing compound' (available from motor shops) with a damp cloth and rub hard. This is a coarse polish which should precede the use of a finer polish such as *T Cut*.

Finally, leave the board to cure at a minimum of 18°C for two weeks.

Appendix IV

Useful Addresses

RYA

Victoria Way, Woking, Surrey.
Tel: 04862 5022.
The Royal Yachting Association acts as the governing body of yachting in the UK. They also organize the Weymouth speed events, and have the responsibility of ratifying all the World Speed Record attempts at other venues.

The RYA also safeguard windsurfers' rights to sail on UK waters; and administers a Funboard course of tuition specifically aimed at short board sailors.

WBA

Feldafinger Platz 2, D8000 Munchen 71, West Germany.
Tel: 089 781074.
The World Boardsailing Association administers the World Cup series of top regattas. The *WBA Rule Book* is invaluable for anyone wanting to organize a serious slalom or wave performance event.

BFA

163 West Lane, Hayling Island, Hants.
Tel: 0705 463595
The British Funboard Association is the principal organizer of national wave and slalom events in the UK.

The British Red Cross Society

9 Grosvenor Crescent, London SW1. The address of your local Red Cross Branch headquarters can be found in the phone book. They provide a variety of First Aid courses which will give you the basic knowledge of how to deal with an emergency on the water or beach.

Appendix V

Sail Materials

Brand Names

Aquaflite
Dutch sailcloth supplier.
Aqualam
GTS laminate sail fabrics.
Cordura
Heavy duty nylon used for luff tubes.
CYT
Howe & Bainbridge hard resin finish woven cloth.
Dacron
Dupont polyester fibre woven cloth.
Dupont
American cloth and chemical company.
GTS
UK manufacturer of sail laminates.
Howe & Bainbridge
Dutch/American sail cloth supplier.
ICI
UK chemical company producing polyester in film and fabric form.
Kevlar
Dupont aramatic polymide with very low stretch characteristics.
LDS
Hard resin finish woven material produced by Ten Cate of Holland.
Melinex
ICI polyester film.
Mylar
Dupont polyester film.

Norlam
North laminated film material.
Plasti Pane
PVC window material.
Polyant
German cloth producer.
Porcher Marine
French cloth producer.
Rip Stop Mylar
Three ply polyester material with rip stop pattern made by Polyant for F2.
Sealam
Porcher Marine laminated fabrics.
Surfkote
Howe & Bainbridge taffeta laminate.
Tejin
Japanese sail cloth producer.
Ten Cate
Dutch sail cloth producer.
Terylene
ICI polyester fibre.
Tetoran
Pryde woven fabric.
Tri Lam
GTS three ply laminate.

Index

Acknowledgments

Jeremy Evans would like to thank the following who have been a particular help with this book: Alex Williams who took most of the photographs; Stuart Sawyer/Astonocean for additional photography and advice on certain advanced techniques; Dave Cordell for advice on aspects of wave riding; Roger Tushingham for help on sail design; Boards Magazine for 'Build Your Own Custom Board'.

Finally, thanks go to Lesley, who helped so much, and to Philip Clark and Julian Holland and their team who edited and designed this book.

Photo Credits
Where not otherwise credited photographs are by Alex Williams.
Stuart Sawyer/Astonocean: pages 14/15, 18/19, 24/25, 26/27, 31, 32, 49, 53, 56/57, 63, 72/73, 80/81, 82/83, 86/87, 88/89, 94/95.
Jeremy Evans: page 29. Sailboard: page 36. Sun Star: pages 38/39. F2: pages 37, 51. Brainwaves: page 41. Fanatic: pages 68/69. Christian Petit: pages 118/119. Vinta: pages 120/121. Bob Barbour: pages 126/127. Paul Carroll: pages 130/131.